618.97

ANGLO-EUROPEA

commitment to medical education.

FOR REFERENCE ONLY

WITHDRAWN FROM
A.E.C.C. LIBRARY

ANGLO-EUROPEAN COLLEGE OF CHIROPRACTIC

Pocket Picture Guides

Geriatrics

Pocket Picture Guides

Geriatrics

Asif Kamal MB BS, MRCP

Consultant Physician in Geriatric Medicine
St. George's Hospital
Lincoln, UK.

Gower Medical Publishing • London • New York • 1986

© Copyright 1986 by Gower Medical Publishing Ltd. 34-42 Cleveland Street, London W1P 5FB, England. All rights reserved. No part of this publication may be reproduced, stored in a retrieval system or transmitted in any form or by any means electronic, mechanical, photocopying, recording or otherwise, without prior written permission of the publisher.

ISBN: 0 906923 67 0

British Library Cataloguing in Publication Data
Kamal, Asif
  Geriatrics. – (Pocket picture guides)
  1. Geriatrics
  I. Title   II. Series
  618.97   RC952

Project Editor: Michele Campbell
  Designer: Sharon Hayles
  Illustrator: Pam Corfield

Printed in Italy by Imago Publishing Ltd.
Set in Baskerville and Univers 45.

Acknowledgements

I wish to express my thanks and gratitude to the people listed below for the loan of their illustrations: Dr. R.O. Barnard (Figs.23 and 38); Boehwinger Ingelheim (Fig.18); Professor P.L. Lantos (Fig.36); Dr. N.I. McNeil (Fig.98); Dr. S. Mejzner (Fig.65); Dr. I. Paterson (Fig.88); Dr. T. Powel (Figs.32, 34 and 63); Dr. H.M. Wisniewski and Churchill Livingstone (Fig.37); Wolfe Medical Publications (Figs.9 and 146).

A.K.
Lincoln

Preface

The aim of this Pocket Picture Guide is to provide the newcomer to the specialty of geriatric medicine with essential visual information about commonly encountered diseases in the elderly. It makes no attempt to cover the whole realm of medicine in old age, but rather illustrates pictorially the fact that the clinical presentation of disease in old age is not only varied but often very different from that in younger patients. Commonly encountered problems such as strokes, dementia and incontinence are presented in individual sections and these include other disorders which may form part of, or contribute to the major syndromes. Medical treatment and geriatric rehabilitation are not included, as these are major subjects and beyond the scope of this book.

I hope that this small book will be of use to all those who have to care for the elderly sick.

A.K.
Lincoln

Contents

Acknowledgements	v
Preface	vi
Introduction	1
Faints and Falls	5
Strokes	11
Brain Failure	19
Pressure Sores	25
Urinary Incontinence	28
Bone Disorders	33
Joint Disorders	41
Cardiovascular Disorders	45
Disorders of the Chest	49
Gastrointestinal Disorders	54
Muscular Disorders	61
Skin Disorders	66
Malignancy in Old Age	72
Miscellaneous Disorders	78
Bibliography	85
Index	

Introduction

Geriatric medicine is a branch of general medicine concerned with the clinical, preventative, remedial and social aspects of health and disease in the elderly. The industrialized countries of the world have experienced a dramatic increase in the number of their elderly. At the beginning of this century, 4.7% of the population of Great Britain was 65 years of age and over. By 1980 the figure had risen to 14.5%. It is predicted that over the next twenty years the number of people who are 75 years of age and over will increase by 20% and indeed in some areas the elderly may constitute up to 40% of the population.

Most patients under the care of geriatric medical departments are over the age of 75. The initial referral is usually with an acute medical illness, superimposed on a background of multiple sociomedical problems. However not every elderly patient is 'geriatric' and similarly not every geriatric patient is over the age of 75.

Medicine in old age is characterized by multiple pathology, altered disease presentation and misleading physical signs. The important aspects of treatment are the concept of whole person medicine and the multidisciplinary team approach to management and rehabilitation.

The cardinal presenting feaures of illness in old age are mental confusion, incontinence, instability and immobility. Each is a symptom which has many different causes and therefore requires a thorough examination and appropriate investigation. The so-called classical features of a particular disease are often absent or modified in elderly patients. The clinician in geriatric medicine knows that misleading or absent physical signs are the hallmark of disease in the elderly and so would not be surprised by a patient with bronchopneumonia presenting with acute confusion, or a case of bacterial endocarditis with only minimal signs.

ANGLO-EUROPEAN COLLEGE OF CHIROPRACTIC

Similarly, loud systolic murmurs may be detected in the absence of significant cardiac disease and Parkinsonism can present without any sign of tremor.

As they grow older, elderly patients tend to develop chronic diseases. Very often the underlying chronic illness is brought to the fore by an unrelated acute disease. Commonly occuring chronic disorders in old age include Parkinsonism, incontinence, glaucoma, osteoarthritis and chronic obstructive airways disease.

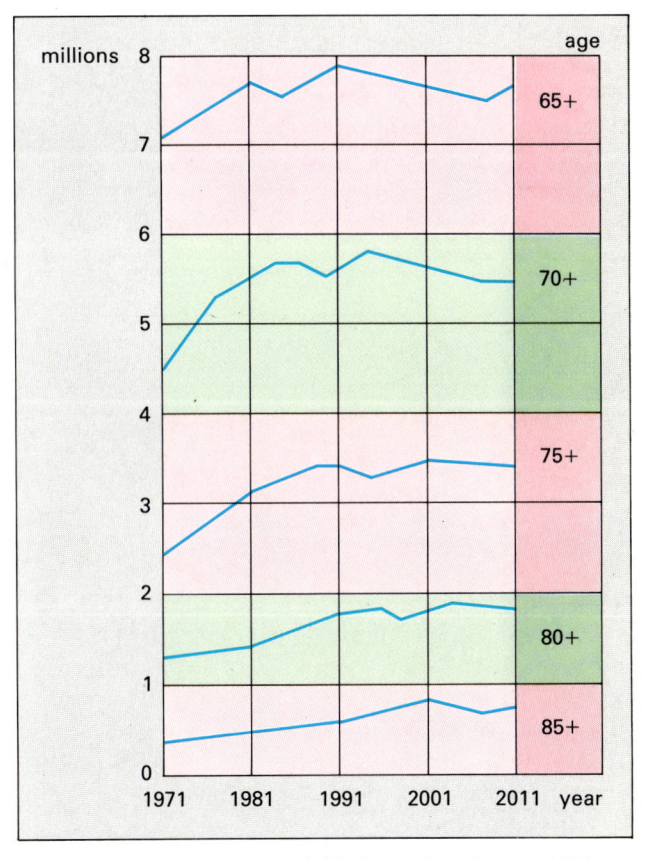

Fig.1 Increase in the number of elderly people to the year 2011.

Department of geriatric medicine	
In patient	**Out patient**
acute assessment wards	day hospital
rehabilitation and continuing care wards	incontinence service
stroke unit	
orthogeriatric unit	home assessment service
unit for elderly mentally disabled (psychogeriatrics)	

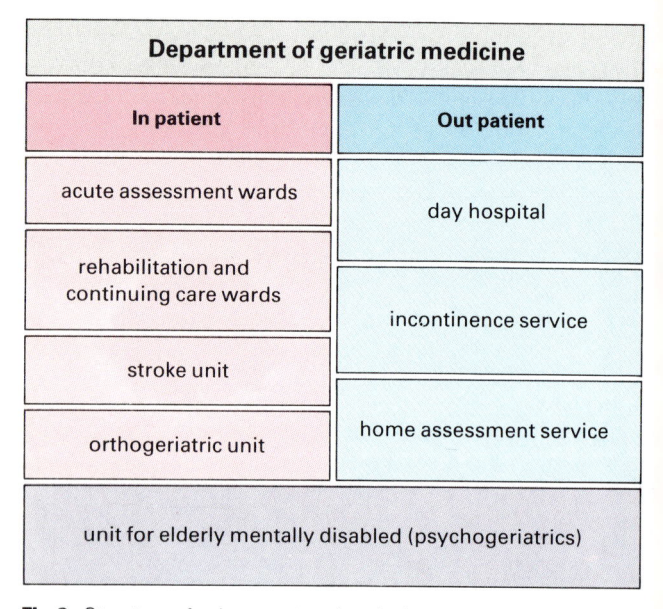

Fig.2 Structure of a department of geriatric medicine.

Multidisciplinary team

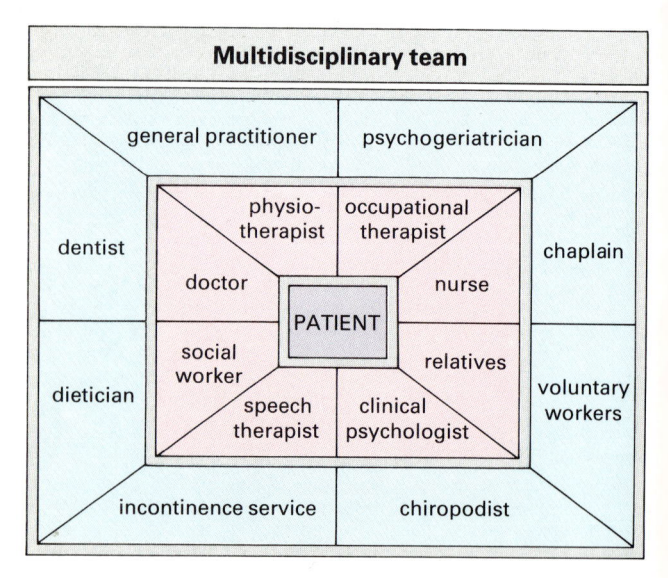

- general practitioner
- psychogeriatrician
- dentist
- chaplain
- dietician
- voluntary workers
- incontinence service
- chiropodist

Inner team around PATIENT:
- physiotherapist
- occupational therapist
- doctor
- nurse
- social worker
- relatives
- speech therapist
- clinical psychologist

Fig.3 Multidisciplinary team for the assessment and rehabilitation of elderly patients.

When examining an elderly patient, one must always consider the normal, age-related changes which are invariably present. If dementia is suspected, a standard mental test should be performed and the primitive reflexes checked. The patient's background should always be included in the overall assessment.

Hazards of minor illness

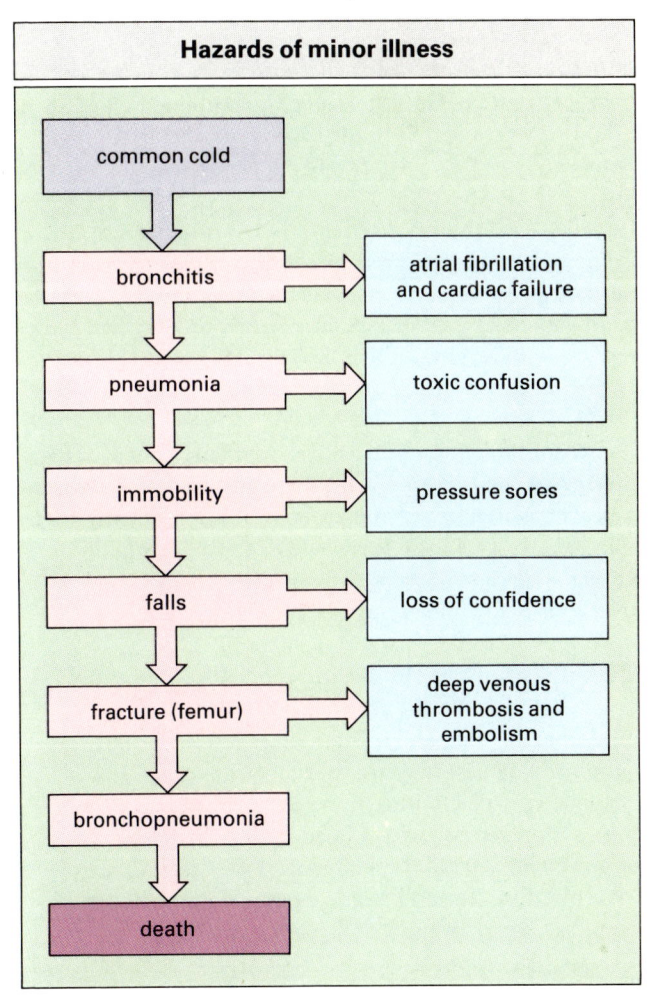

common cold → bronchitis → pneumonia → immobility → falls → fracture (femur) → bronchopneumonia → death

- bronchitis → atrial fibrillation and cardiac failure
- pneumonia → toxic confusion
- immobility → pressure sores
- falls → loss of confidence
- fracture (femur) → deep venous thrombosis and embolism

Fig.4 Hazards of minor illness in elderly patients.

Faints and Falls

Faints and falls are common in elderly patients. The incidence increases with age and they are more frequent in women who are socially isolated, depressed or disabled. They may be caused by a wide variety of disorders ranging from ill-fitting footwear to drop attacks. The latter occur in patients suffering from a combination of cervical spine arthritis and atheroma of the vertebral arteries. They occur without loss of consciousness or neurological sequelae but the patient is frequently unable to stand afterwards unless helped. About 12-25% of falls in the elderly are due to drop attacks.

Cardiac arrhythmias, particularly heart block, are frequently responsible for instability in the elderly. A patient whose cerebral circulation is already compromised by atheroma may faint if any further reduction in cerebral blood flow occurs due to the onset of cardiac arrhythmia.

Parkinsonian patients also have a tendency to fall. This is due to a combination of restricted mobility, increased muscle rigidity, poor balance, postural hypotension and the side effects of drug therapy. Other causes of faints and falls include backward sway, osteoarthritis and transient ischaemic attacks.

The most common complications of falls in the elderly are fractures (especially of the wrist and femur), extensive bruising and head injuries. Of the latter, subdural haematomas are the most frequent, and can occur after even a minor injury to the head. All elderly patients presenting with a head injury should be observed for several days afterwards and the investigations should include a plain X-ray of the skull, an ultrasound scan and a CT scan if available.

Causes of faints and falls in the elderly

Enviromental and accidental

slippery surfaces
narrow, steep stairs

Lower limb abnormalities

bunions, warts and corns
oedema of the feet
hallux valgus, hammer toes
osteoarthritis of hip
peripheral vascular disease
onychogryphosis

Neurological disorders

TIAs
epilepsy
Parkinsonism
strokes-in-evolution
cerebellar disorders
brain tumours

Cardiovascular disorders

silent myocardial infarction
arrhythmias
postural hypotension
subclavian steal syndrome
severe anaemias

Drop attacks

Miscellaneous

carotid sinus hypersensitivity
micturition syncope
loss of confidence
drugs (hypnotics)
visual impairment
vasovagal attacks
defaecation syncope
hypoglycaemia
osteomalacia

Fig.5 Causes of faints and falls in the elderly.

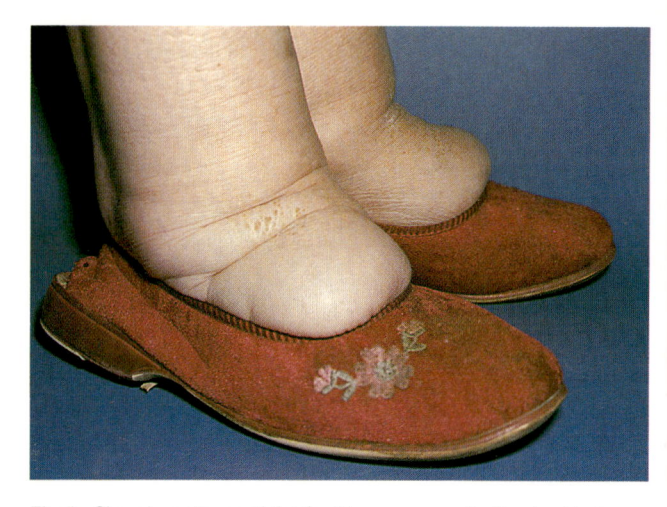

Fig.6 Chronic oedema of the feet is a common finding in elderly patients, especially in those who have limited mobility. Bad sitting posture, gravitation and venous insufficiency contribute to produce such oedema. The loss of the normal contours of the feet causes instability and falls.

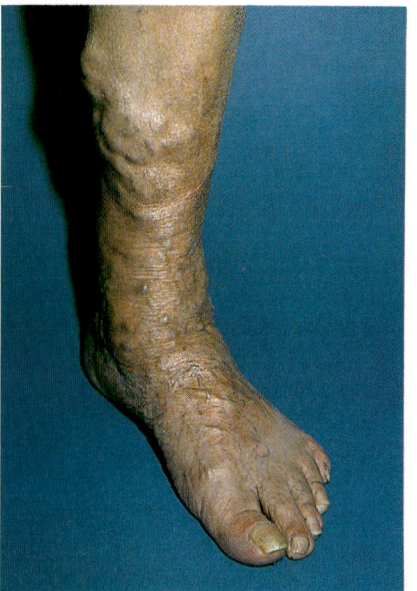

Fig.7 Varicose veins and venous insufficiency in a case of postural hypotension. This condition is one of the commonest causes of falls in the elderly. It is defined as a fall in systolic blood pressure greater than 20mmHg with symptoms of dizziness, faints or falls.

Drop-attacks

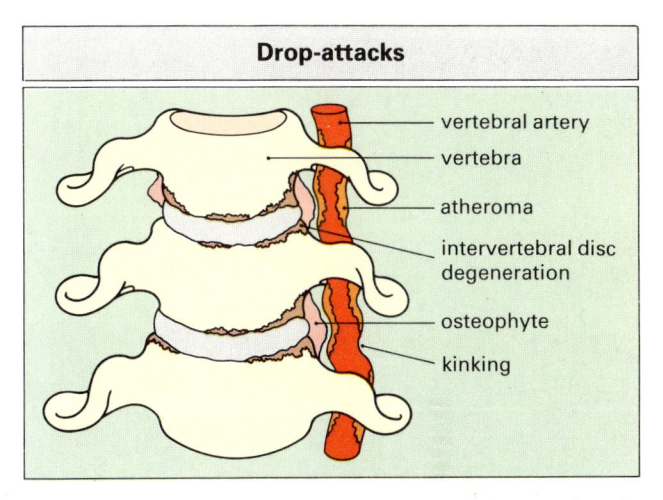

Fig.8 Drop attacks. Cervical spine arthritis causes degeneration of the spine which allows kinking in the atheromatous vertebral artery. A rapid neck movement may cause the osteophytes to impinge on the vertebral artery. If this occurs at the site of an atheromatous plaque, the lumen is temporarily blocked, producing transient ischaemia and resulting in a sudden fall.

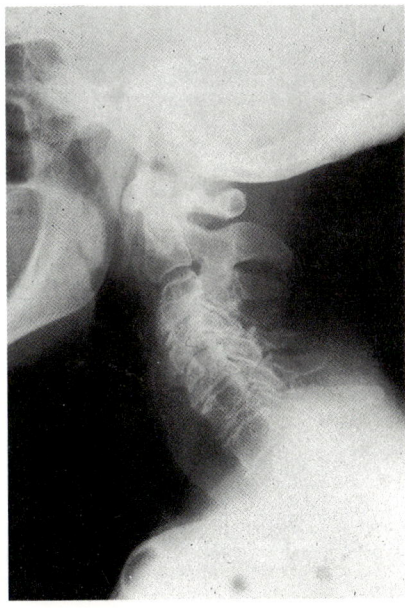

Fig.9 X-ray of the cervical spine showing advance degenerative changes, with slight anterior displacement of C1 on C2.

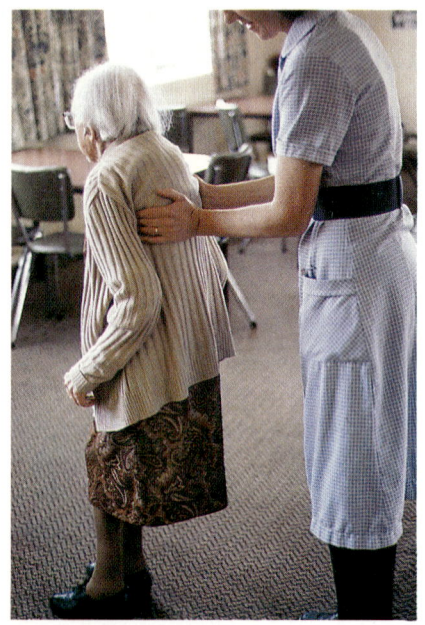

Fig.10 A tendency to sway backwards and fall is a common phenomenon in the elderly. It is due to a disturbance in the central balance mechanism and can occur in a wide variety of illnesses.

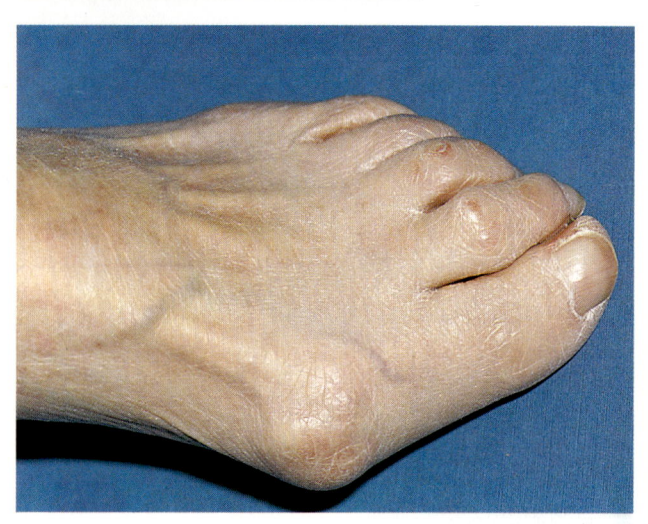

Fig.11 Hallux valgus is a common orthopaedic problem in the elderly. The first metatarsophalangeal joint is prominent with bony enlargement of the inner side of the first metatarsal head. Bilateral hallux valgus interferes with mobility and is a frequent cause of falls.

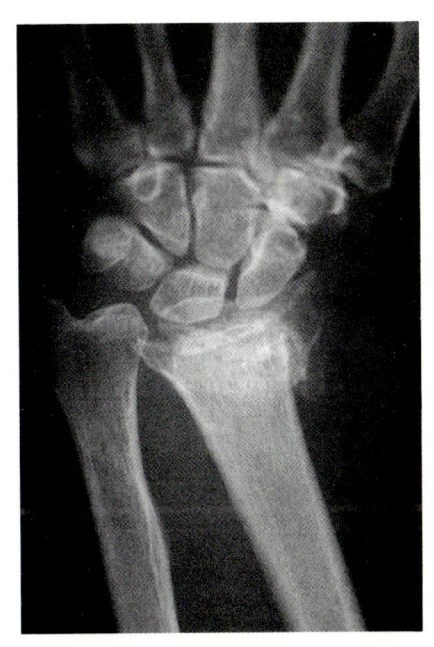

Fig.12 X-ray of the wrist showing a Colles fracture, a frequent complication of falls in old people.

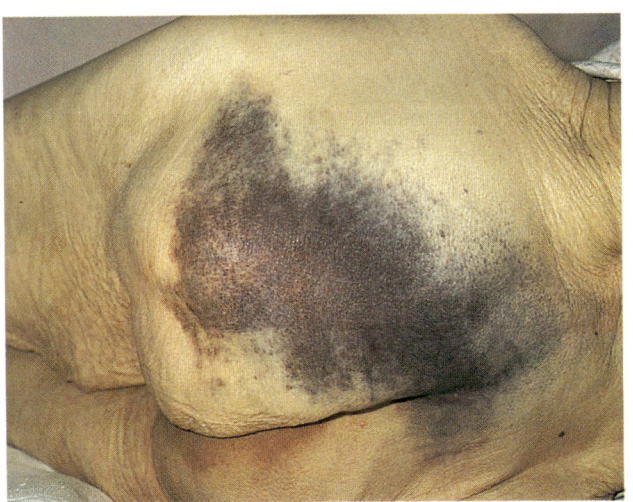

Fig.13 Painful, extensive bruising often results from falls in elderly patients.

Strokes

A stroke is characterized by a focal neurological deficit due to a local disturbance in the blood supply to the brain. Its onset is abrupt but it may extend over a few hours or more. Atheroma and hypertension are the principal pathogenetic factors in cerebrovascular disease. Atherothromboembolic brain infarction accounts for about 80% of all strokes.

Complications of strokes
pressure sores
respiratory infections
urinary incontinence
deep vein thrombosis
spasticity and contractures
frozen shoulder
psychiatric problems
shoulder-hand syndrome
recurrent falls

Fig.14 Complications of strokes.

Circle of Willis

- anterior cerebral artery
- middle cerebral artery
- posterior cerebral artery
- basilar artery
- pontine arteries
- anterior inferior cerebellar artery
- vertebral artery
- posterior inferior cerebellar artery
- ● common sites of atheroma

Fig.15 Circle of Willis showing common sites of atheroma.

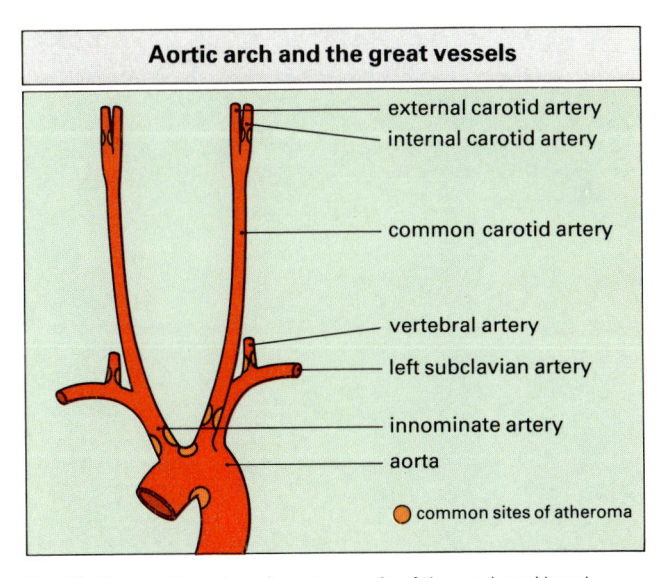

Aortic arch and the great vessels

- external carotid artery
- internal carotid artery
- common carotid artery
- vertebral artery
- left subclavian artery
- innominate artery
- aorta
- ● common sites of atheroma

Fig.16 The aortic arch and great vessels of the neck and head showing common sites of atheroma.

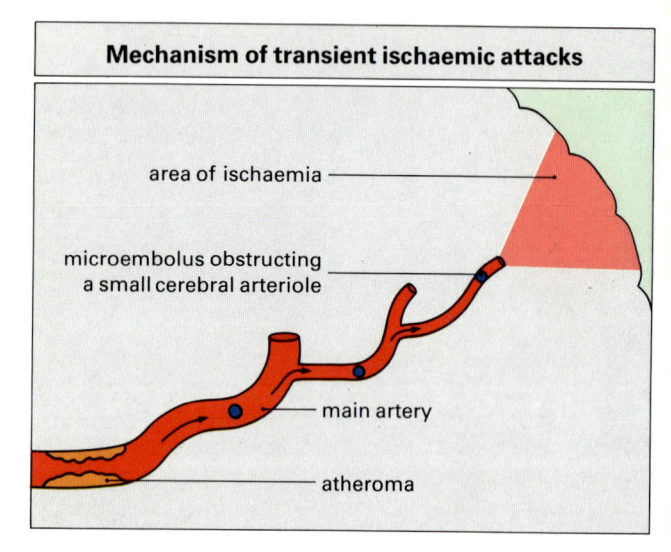

Fig. 17 Transient ischaemic attack (TIA). This is an acute episode of focal neurological or retinal dysfunction lasting less then 24 hours. TIAs are due to microemboli arising from the heart or carotid artery and lodging in the small cerebral blood vessels. About one third of patients go on to develop a major stroke.

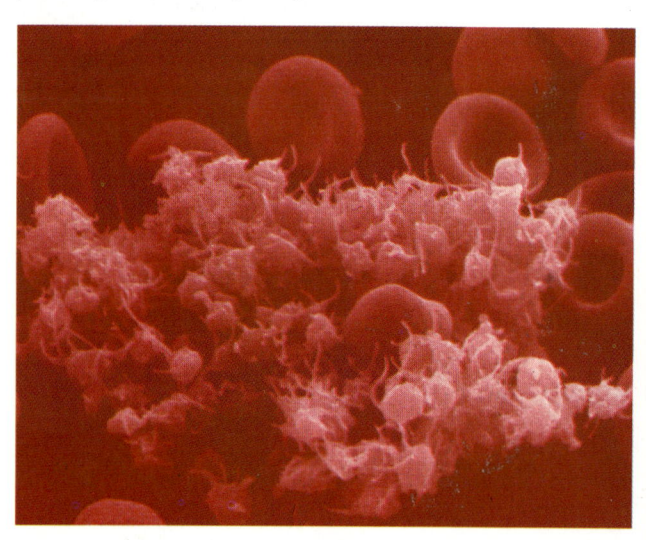

Fig. 18 Scanning electron micrograph of a platelet microembolus, the cause of TIAs.

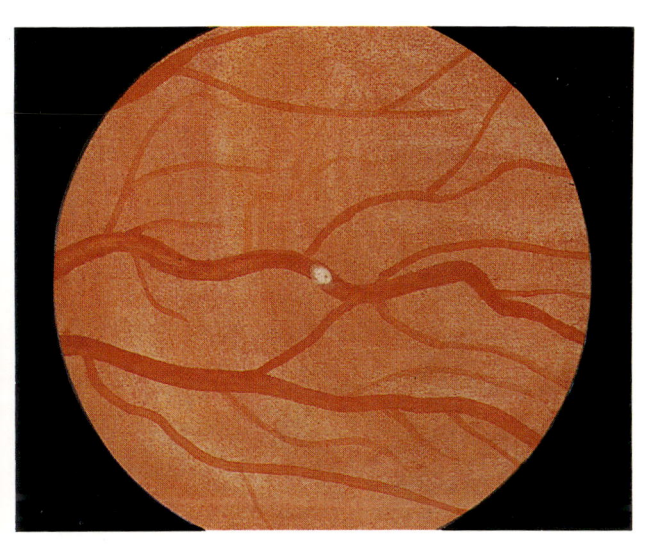

Fig.19 A cholesterol embolus in a retinal blood vessel giving rise to amaurosis fugax.

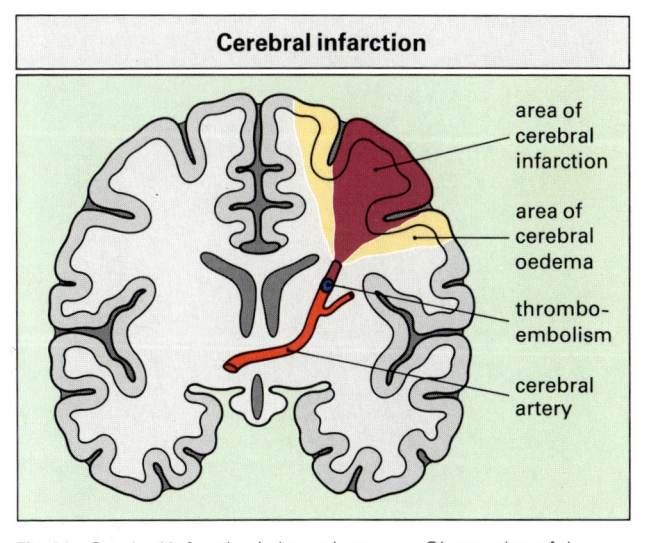

Fig.20 Cerebral infarction in its early stages. Obstruction of the artery leads to the development of a discrete area of cerebral infarction. The subsequent oedematous reaction around the infarcted tissue causes further cerebral damage. This can be restricted by early, intensive medical management.

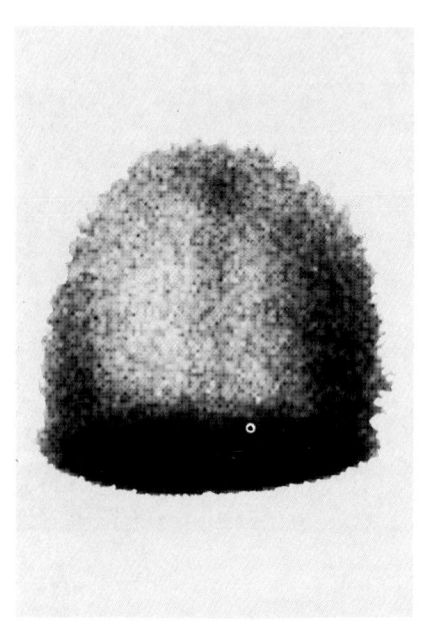

Fig.21 Isotope brain scan showing large areas of increased uptake in the parietal and occipital regions of the left hemisphere. This elderly patient presented with right hemiplegia and aphasia.

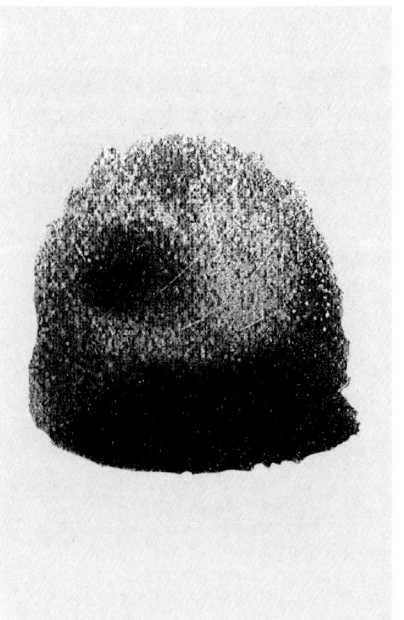

Fig.22 Isotope brain scan showing a large tumour in the right hemisphere. The patient presented with signs of left hemiparesis and personality changes.

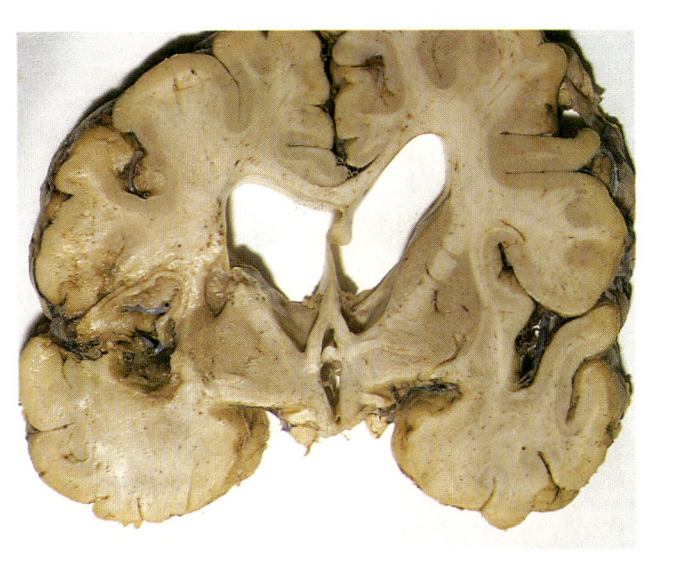

Fig.23 This brain was removed from an 81-year-old patient and shows enlarged ventricles and an infarct.

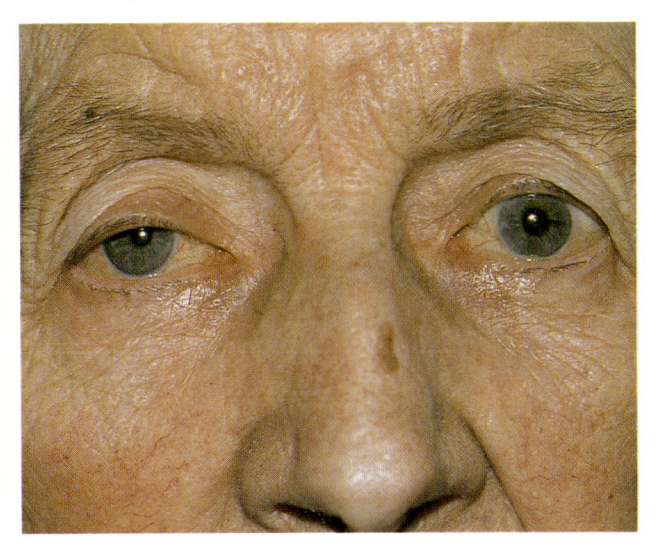

Fig.24 Right-sided ptosis due to a cerebrovascular accident. This is a frequent finding in elderly patients. Its causes include vascular lesions, tumours, congenital third nerve palsy, multiple sclerosis and myasthenia gravis.

Visual field defects

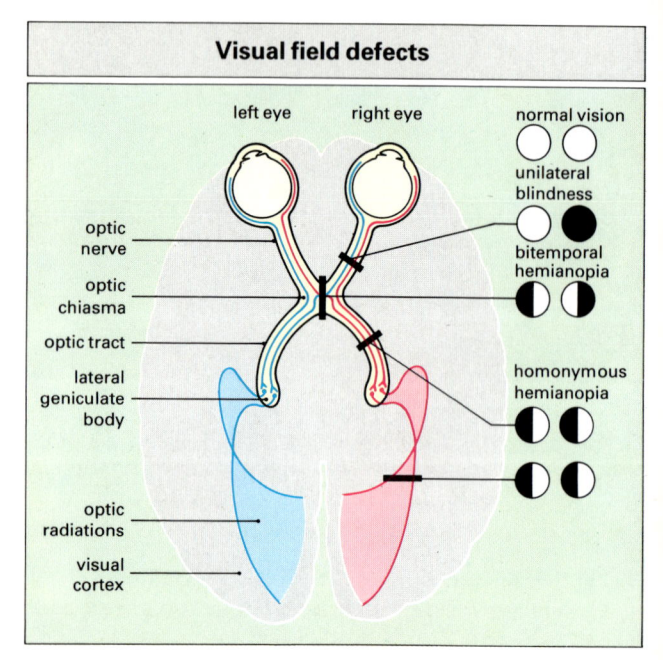

Fig.25 The effect on the field of vision produced by lesions at various points along the optic pathway. Hemianopia is commonly associated with cerebral infarction. If the vascular lesion involves the optic tract or the visual cortex, homonymous hemianopia will result.

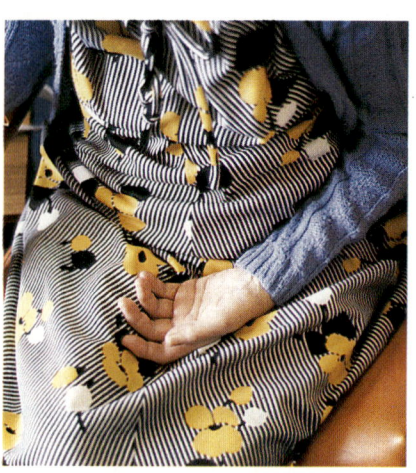

Fig.26 Typical posture of the left hand due to hemiplegic paralysis.

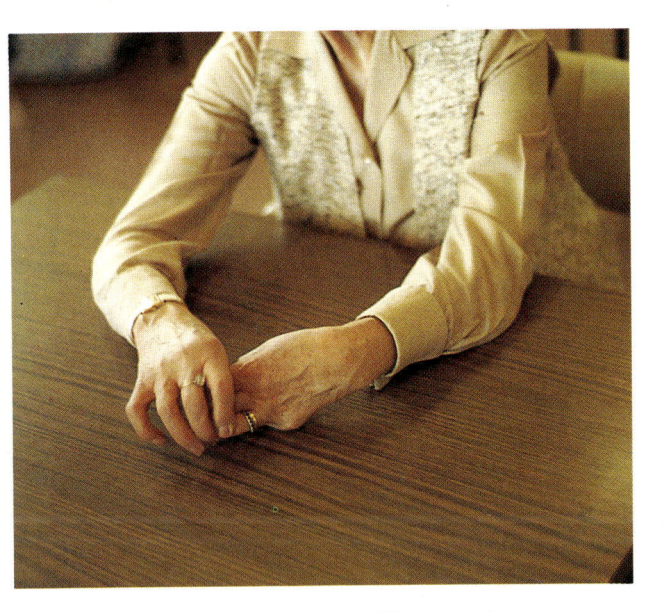

Fig.27 Flaccid paralysis of the left arm. This can lead to shoulder subluxation if the arm is allowed to hang unsupported.

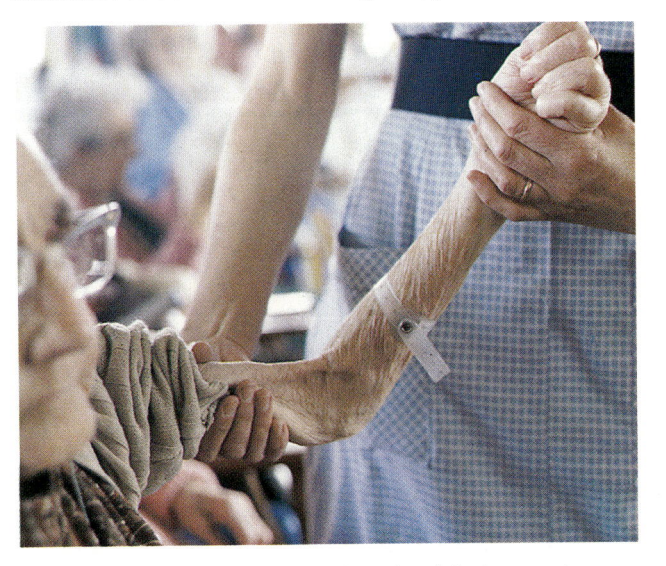

Fig.28 Contracture of the left arm due to hemiplegia several years previously.

Brain Failure
(Confusional States and Dementia)

Mental confusion is one of the commonest presenting symptoms of illness in old age. A reduced reserve of cortical neurones allows acute illnesses, which normally produce anoxia and toxaemia, to overcome the limited cerebral function and present as confusion. Dementia, however, appears gradually and runs a prolonged course. It presents as diffuse impairment of the intellect and personality, is of insidious onset and is usually progressive.

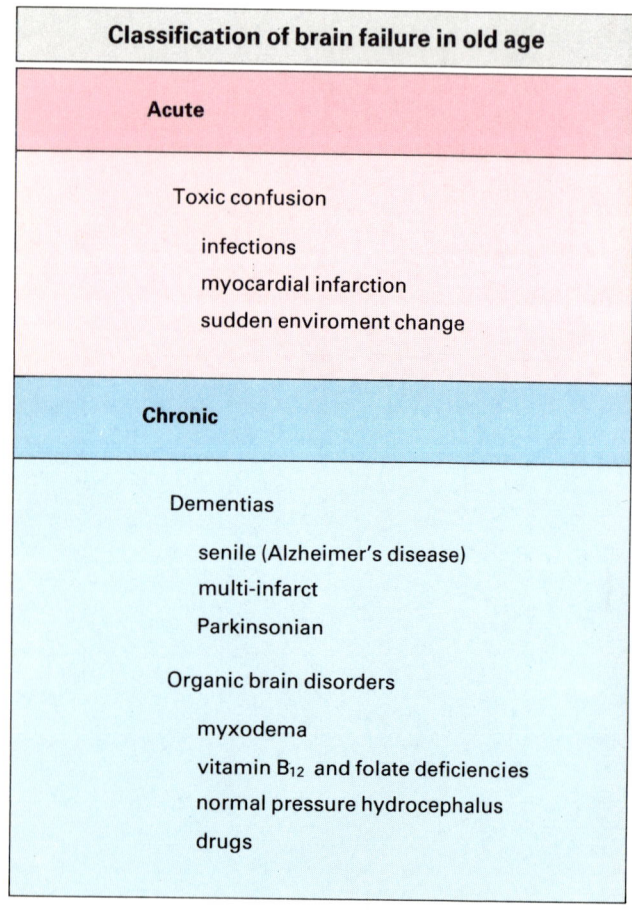

Classification of brain failure in old age
Acute

Toxic confusion
    infections
    myocardial infarction
    sudden enviroment change

Chronic

Dementias
    senile (Alzheimer's disease)
    multi-infarct
    Parkinsonian
Organic brain disorders
    myxodema
    vitamin B_{12} and folate deficiencies
    normal pressure hydrocephalus
    drugs

Fig.29 Classification of brain failure in old age.

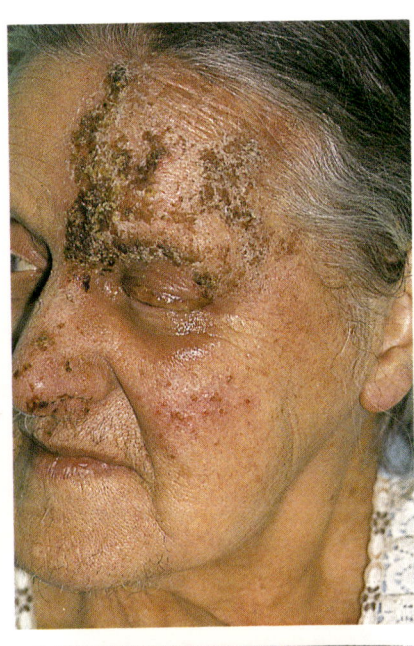

Fig.30 Ophthalmic herpes zoster presenting with pain, agitation and acute confusion.

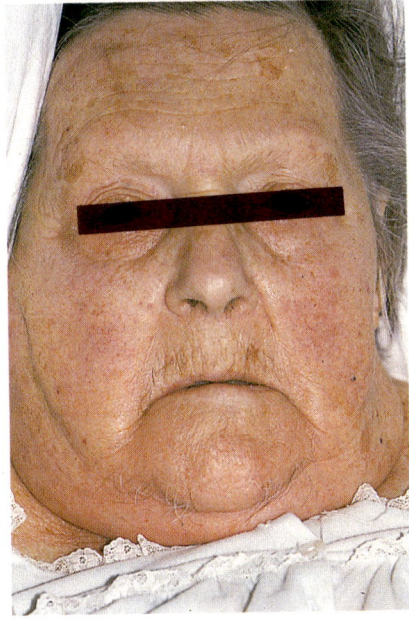

Fig.31 Steroid-induced dementia. This patient had developed secondary Cushing's syndrome and increasing dementia due to prolonged use of corticosteroids for chronic rheumatoid arthritis.

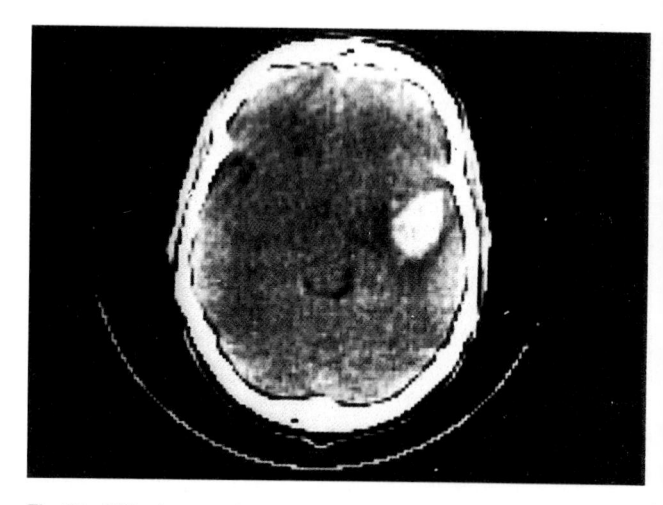

Fig.32 CT brain scan showing a temporal lobe haematoma due to a middle cerebral artery aneurysm. The patient presented with hemiplegia and confusion.

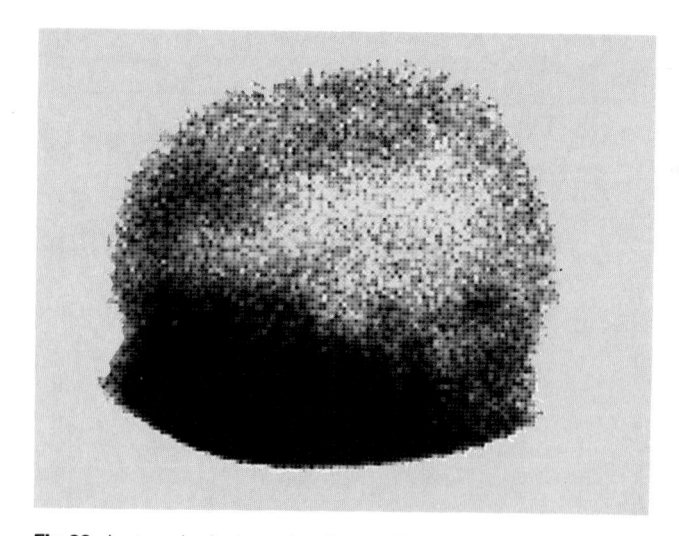

Fig.33 Isotope brain scan showing multiple areas of increased uptake. The patient had suffered a number of strokes over a period of years and showed signs of multi-infarct dementia including personality alteration, restlessness and paranoia. Physically, the patient showed increasing rigidity, shuffling gait and falls.

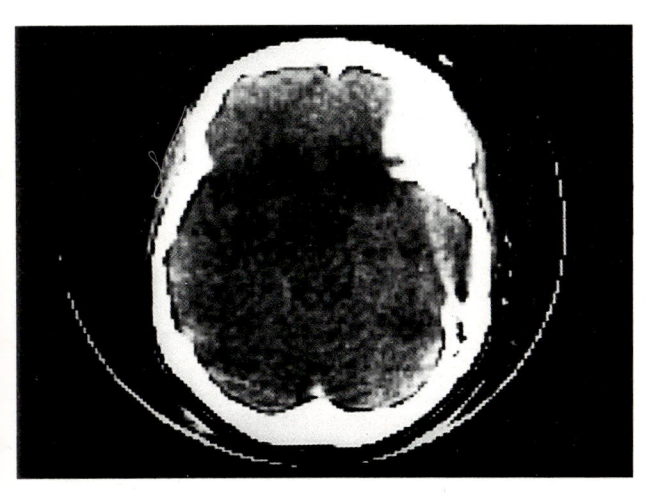

Fig.34 CT brain scan showing bony hyperostosis of the skull secondary to a meningioma. Patients with this tumour frequently present with dementia. It is important to diagnose the condition, as early surgery can be curative.

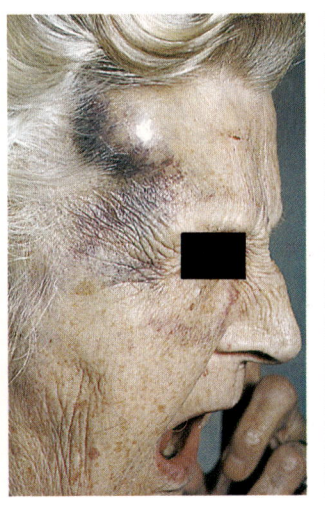

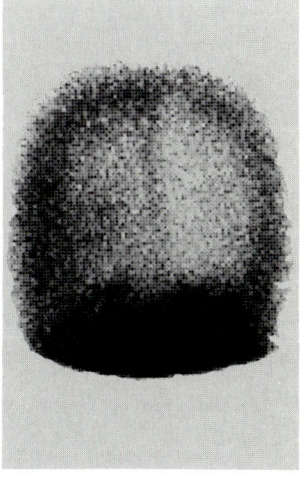

Fig.35 This patient suffered an accidental fall resulting in mild bruising and swelling over the right temple (left). X-rays of the skull did not show any bony injury. Weeks later she began to behave abnormally and presented with confusion, unsteadiness, lethargy and headaches. An isotope brain scan (right) showed the presence of a large subdural haematoma.

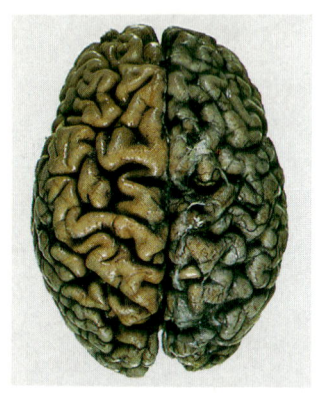

Fig.36 This brain was taken from a patient who presented with the clinical features of advanced senile dementia. It shows marked general atrophy with shrunken gyri and gaping sulci.

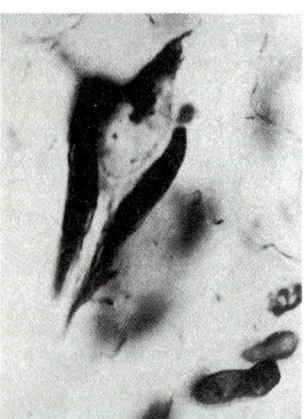

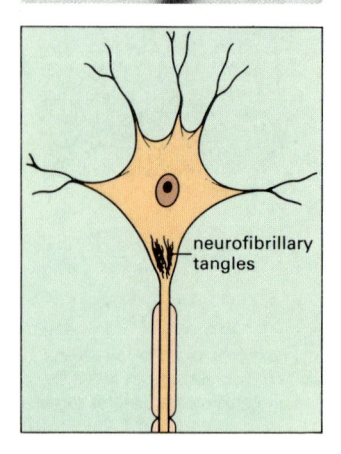

Fig.37 One of the typical histological features of senile dementia is the presence of neurofibrillary tangles (top) which consist of degenerated neurofilaments. They are intraneuronal, situated towards the periphery of the cell at the axon hillock (bottom).

neurofibrillary tangles

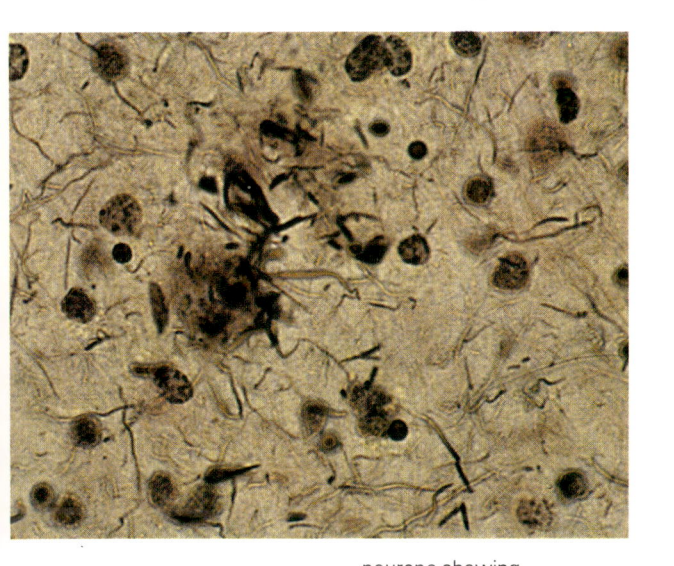

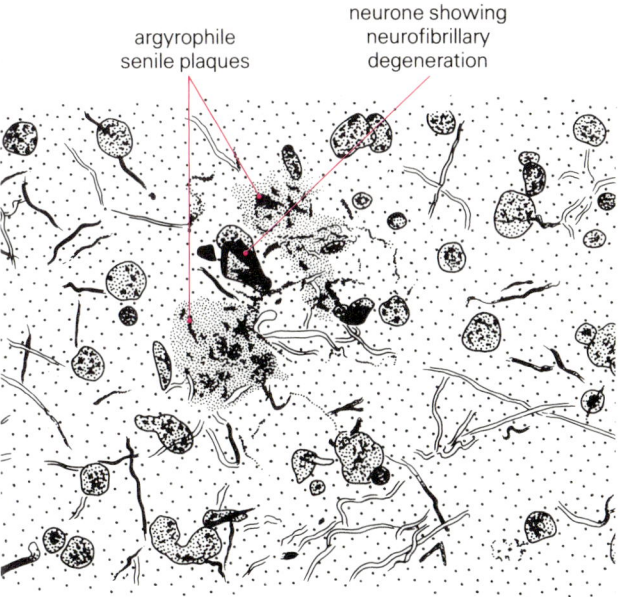

Fig.38 Senile plaques are also typical histological features of senile dementia. They consist of a central amyloid core surrounded by degenerating mitochondria, lysosomes and macrophages, and are widespread in the grey matter.

Pressure Sores

Pressures sores were once a common problem in patients who had to remain immobile for prolonged periods. Now, however, with modern nursing techniques and the availability of pressure relieving devices, their incidence is on the decline. There are two main types: superficial, where the prognosis is good with early active treatment; and deep, where tissue necrosis is present and the prognosis is poor. Compression and shearing forces

Pressure sores				
General condition	good	0	fair	1
	poor	2	bad	3
Mental state	alert	0	confused	1
	apathetic	2	stuporous	3
Activity	ambulant	0	needs help	1
	chairfast	2	bedfast	3
Mobility	full	0	decreased	1
	very limited	2	immobile	3
Incontinence	none	0	occasional	1
	incontinent of urine	2	doubly incontinent	3

Fig.39 Exton-Smith's clinical score is used to identify patients who are likely to develop pressure sores. Those scoring over 7 points are considered to be at risk.

between the patient's body and the supporting surface are the main initiating factors in the development of a pressure sore. Contributory factors include poor tissue perfusion, immobility and paresis and urinary and faecal incontinence.

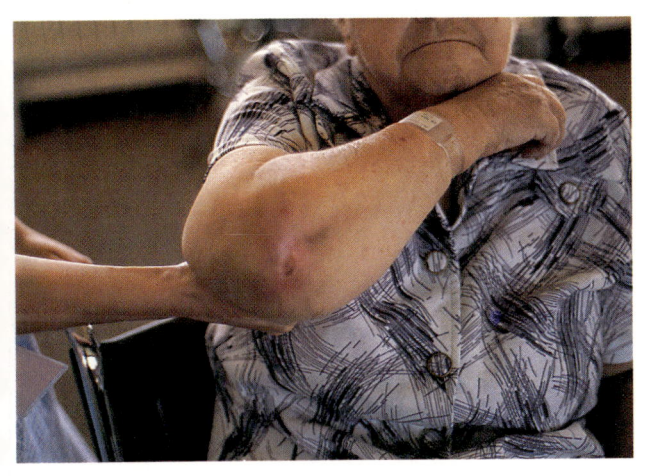

Fig.40 Some pressure sores are brought about by repeated rubbing of vulnerable bony prominences across the bedsheets by confused, restless patients. These sores are also called friction burns.

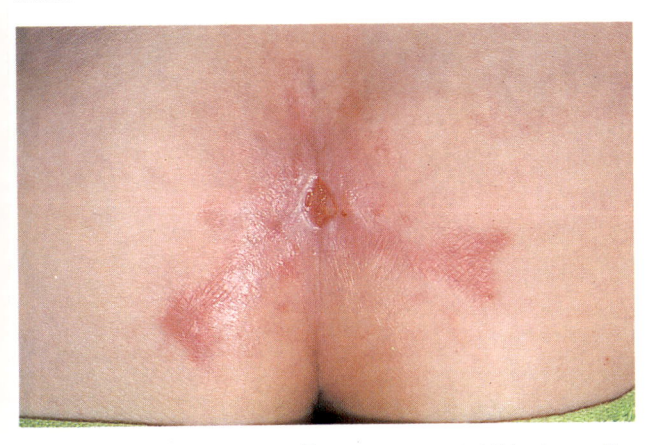

Fig.41 An early pressure sore. Prompt treatment at this stage will halt further deterioration.

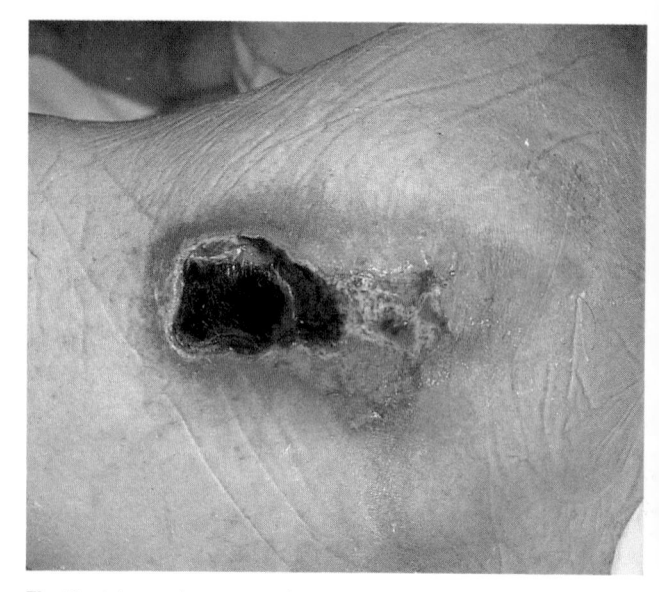

Fig.42 A large, deep, necrotic pressure sore over the hip.

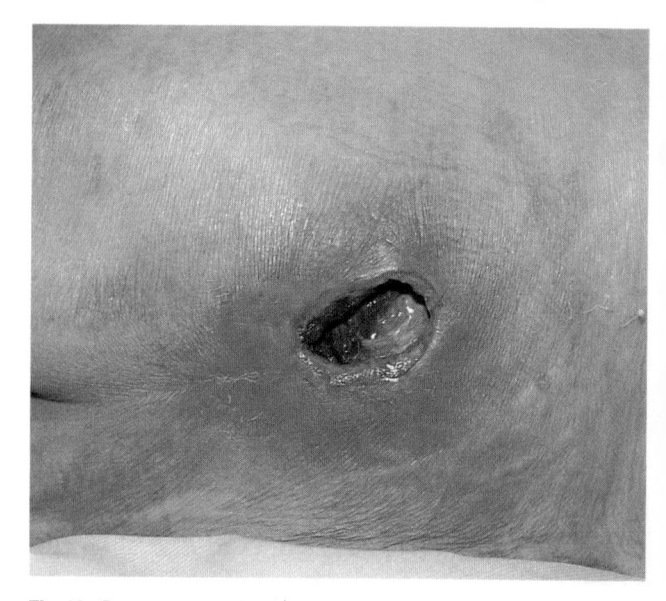

Fig.43 Pressure sore that is gradually healing. Note the appearance of the new skin around the edges of the sore.

Urinary Incontinence

The incidence of urinary incontinence in the elderly may be up to 20-30%.

Aetiology of urinary incontinence

Transient incontinence (treatable)

- urinary tract infections
- retention with infections
- retention with overflow
- increased diuresis
- toxic confusion
- urethral caruncle
- sudden change of environment

Established incontinence

- loss of cortical inhibition
  - dementias,
  - cerebrovascular disorders
- prostatic disease
- bladder stone or carcinoma
- pelvic tumour
- unstable bladder
- spinal cord lesion
- atonic neurogenic bladder
- uterovaginal prolapse

Fig.44 Aetiology of urinary incontinence.

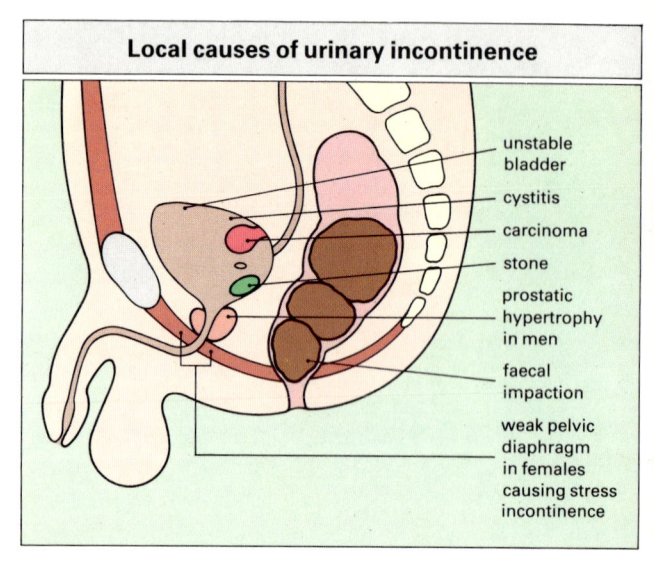

Fig.45 Local causes of urinary incontinence. Prostatic hypertrophy leads to chronic retention with overflow incontinence.

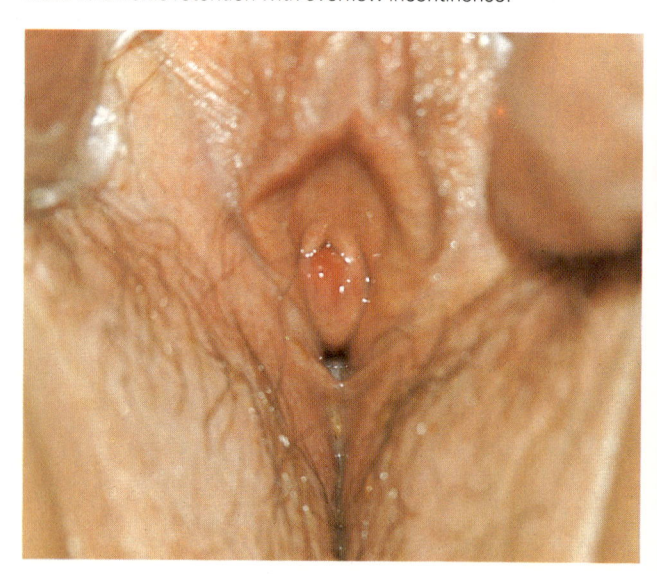

Fig.46 Caruncle. This is the granulomatous end stage of a urethrocele and is a frequent cause of incontinence. This patient also has atrophic vaginitis.

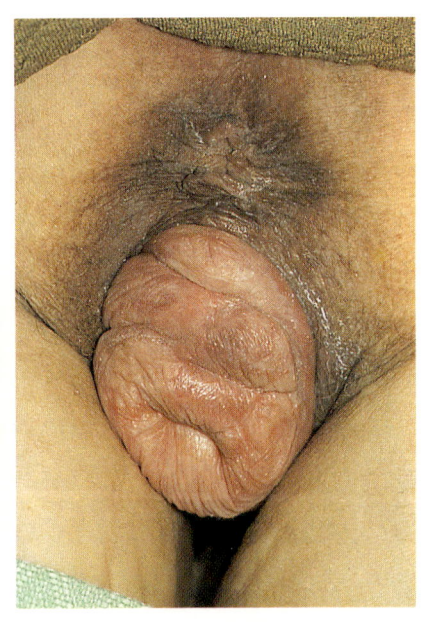

Fig.47 Uterovaginal prolapse is due to a combination of vaginal atrophy, weakness of the vaginal walls and ageing skeletal muscles.

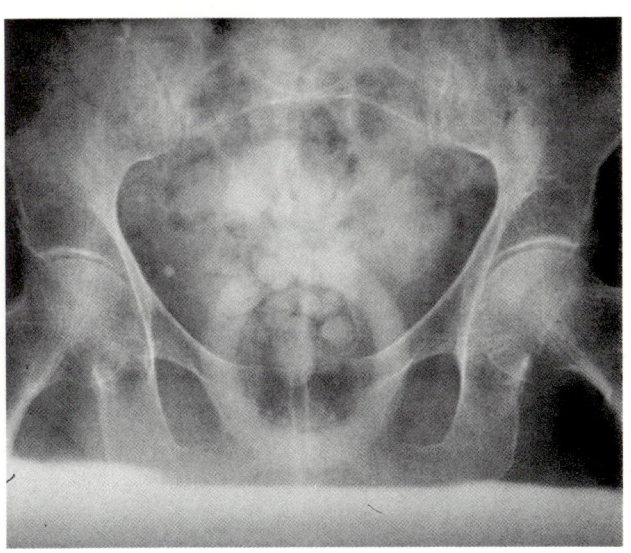

Fig.48 A forgotten ring pessary can give rise to pelvic problems, including incontinence, many years later.

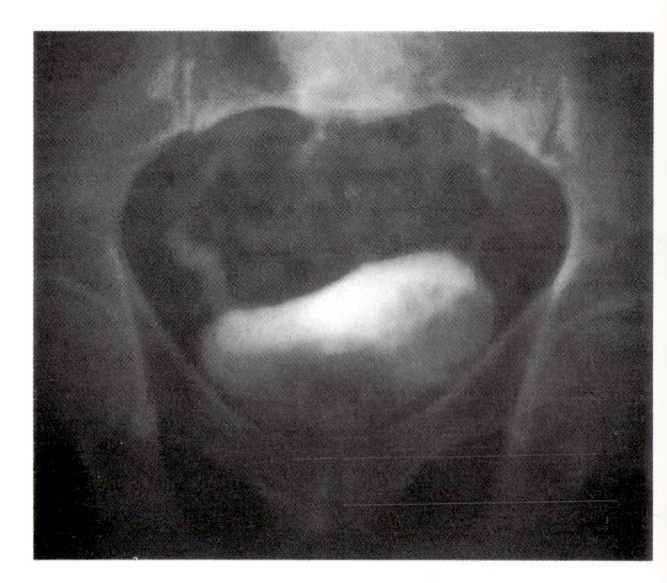

Fig.49 Filling defect at the base of the bladder due to prostatic hypertrophy. This patient also has a papilloma on the left wall of the bladder.

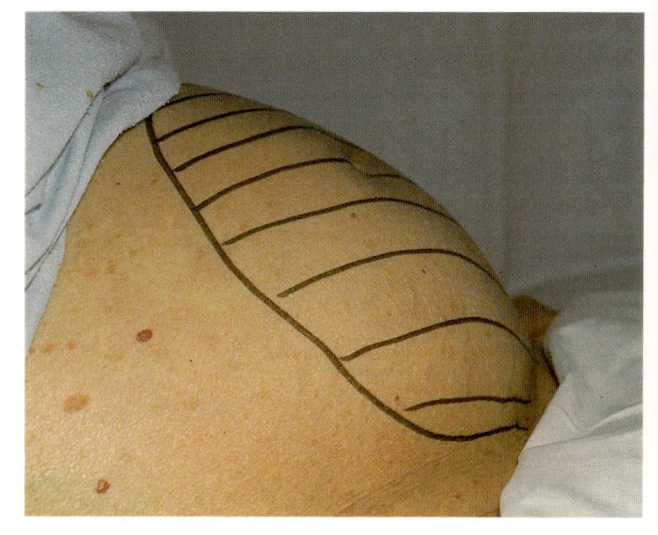

Fig.50 Gross distention of the bladder due to urinary retention, secondary to anticholinergic drugs.

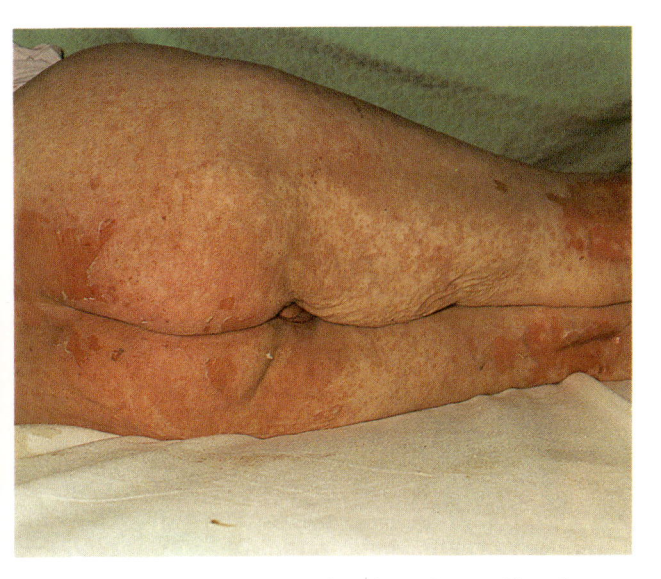

Fig.51 A severe rash caused by urinary incontinence. There is excoriation, cellulitis and early pressure sores are developing.

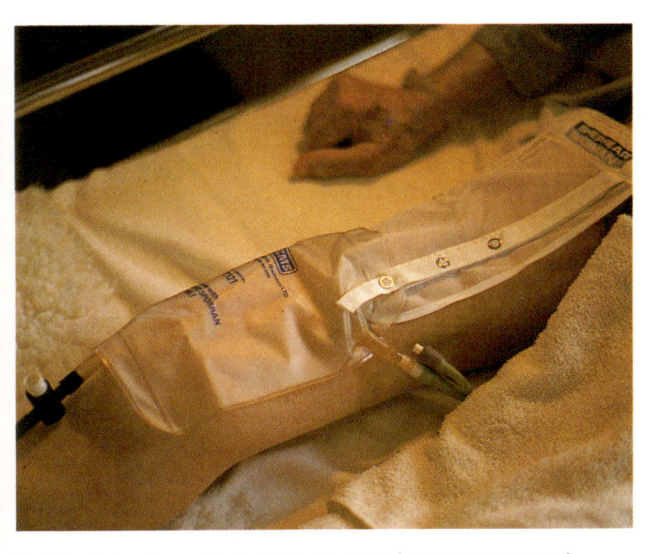

Fig.52 Indwelling catheter with a leg bag for management of intractable incontinence. The bag is slim and can be worn under the clothing, giving the patient confidence and allowing normal mobility.

Bone Disorders

The common bone disorders in old age are fractures (especially of the neck of the femur), osteoporosis, osteomalacia, Paget's disease and metastatic bone diseases. In osteoporosis, the amount of bone per unit volume of bony tissue is reduced. The bones become fragile and fractures occur with minimal trauma. Osteomalacia is characterized by a defect in bone mineralization (often associated with vitamin D deficiency) and an excess of osteoid tissue. These two conditions often occur in the same patient and exact differentiation may be impossible. In Paget's disease, the bone architecture is typically abnormal, due to a defect in the rate of both breakdown and formation of bony tissue. The skull, pelvis, lumbar spine, femur and tibia are the most commonly affected sites and the incidence tends to be higher in men than women.

Fractures of the neck of the femur

- subcapital
- transcervical
- intertrochanteric
- subtrochanteric

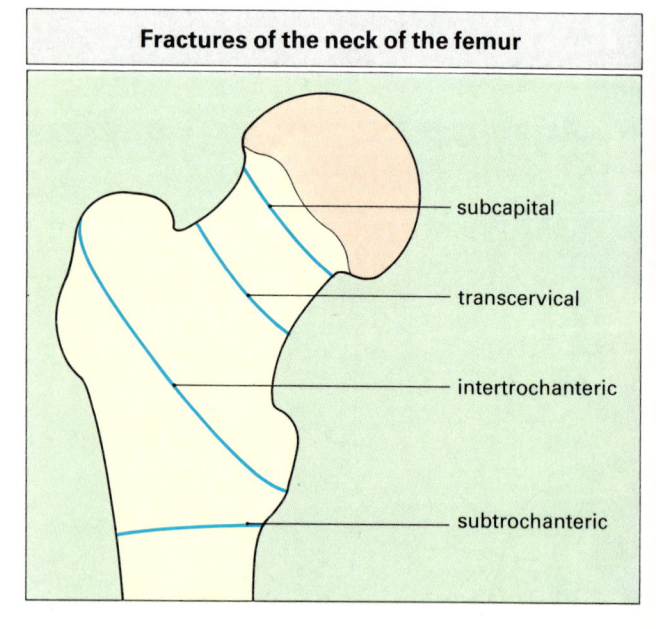

Fig.53 Different types of fracture in the upper end of the femur. This is a common problem in elderly people. Fracture of the neck of the femur occurs most frequently, usually after a fall in a patient with osteoporosis.

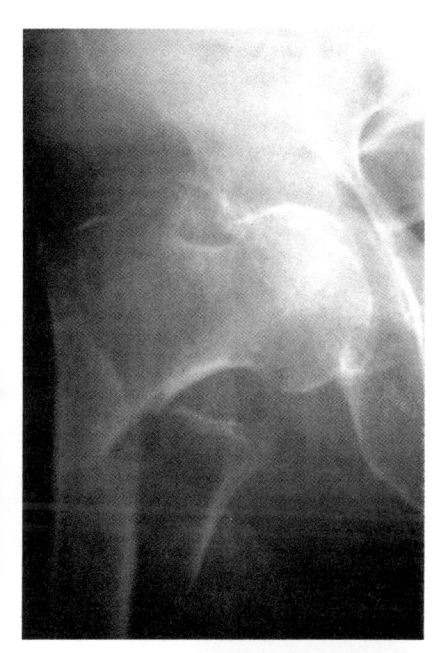

Fig.54 An intertrochanteric fracture (top) of the right hip. An X-ray of the left hip in a different patient shows a subcapital fracture (bottom).

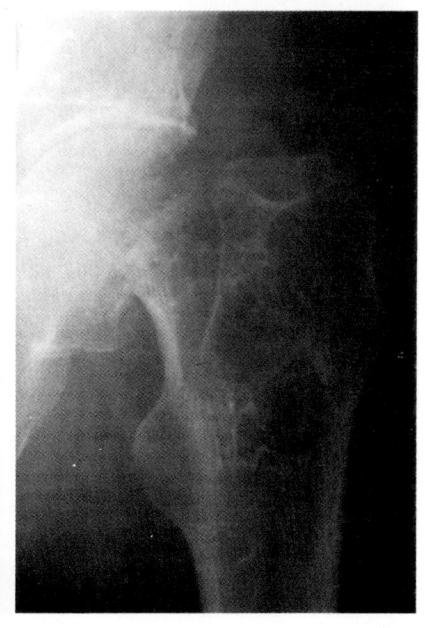

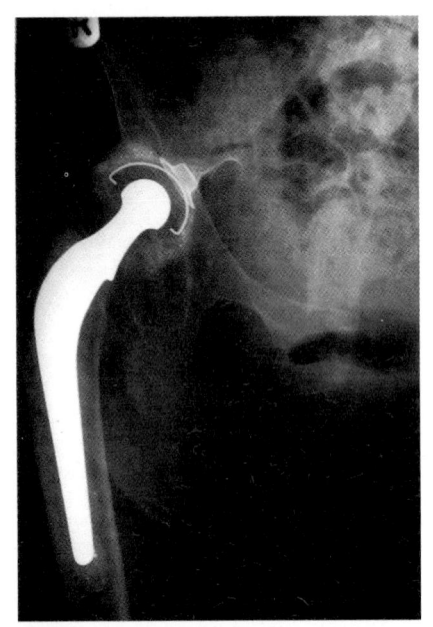

Fig.55 Fracture of the neck of the femur may be treated with Thompson's prosthesis (top) or with a nail and plate (bottom).

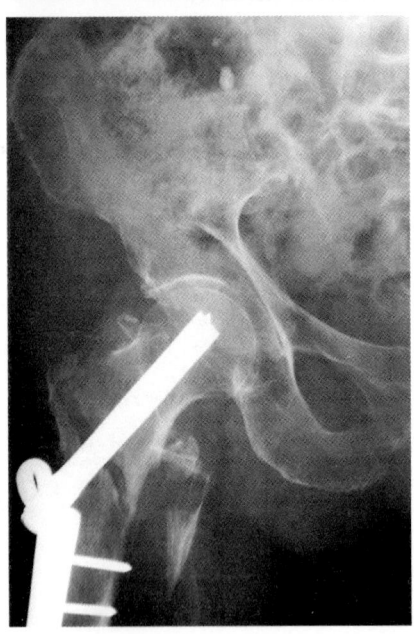

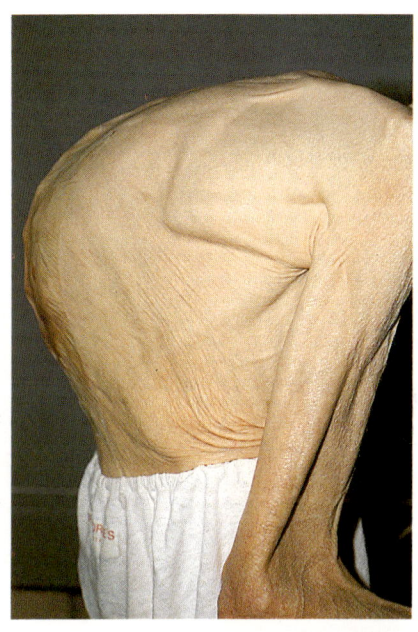

Fig.56 Marked kyphosis of the dorsal spine due to multiple osteoporotic fractures of the vertebral bodies. Deformity of the spine may progress slowly, sometimes in the absence of back pain.

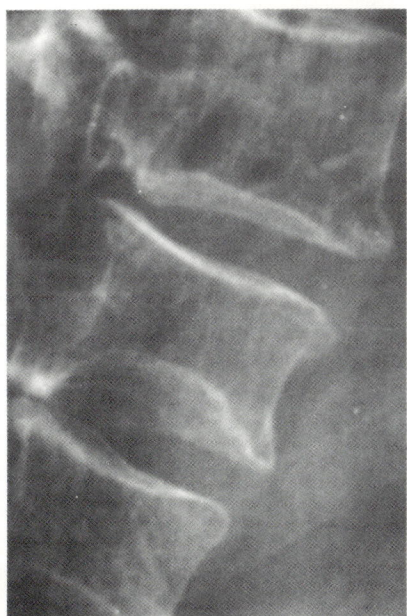

Fig.57 X-ray of the spine showing development of a typical Schmorl's node. This is a sign of advanced osteoporosis, in which there is herniation of the intervertebral disc into the body of the osteoporotic vertebra.

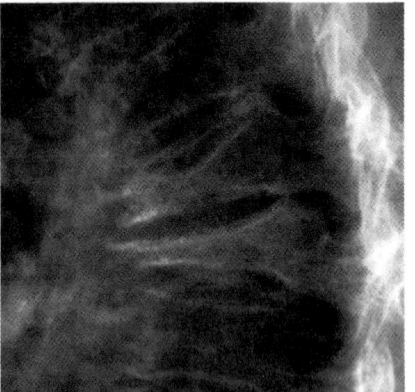

Fig.58 A typical osteoporotic spine showing multiple compression fractures of vertebral bodies (top). The tibia and fibula also show osteoporotic fractures (bottom).

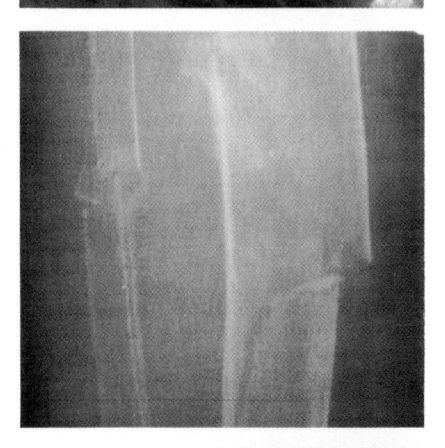

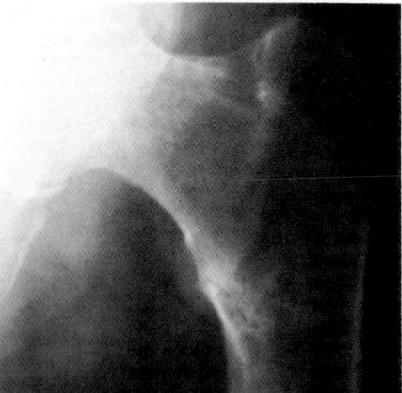

Fig.59 Looser's zone (pseudofracture) in the upper end of the left femur. These are incomplete stress fractures in which the normal process of healing is impaired by the mineralization defect. They may progress to complete fractures.

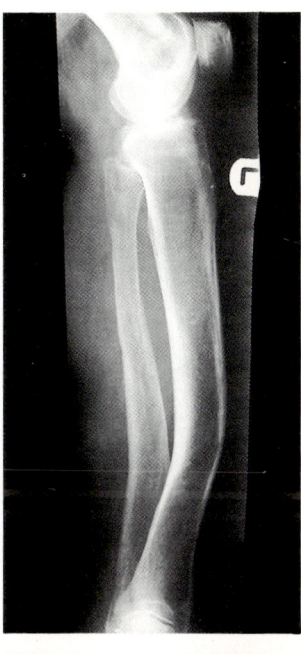

Fig.60 X-ray of the left leg showing bowing of the tibia and fibula. This elderly lady was admitted with depression and immobility. She was found to have osteomalacia and made a dramatic improvement after treatment with vitamin D.

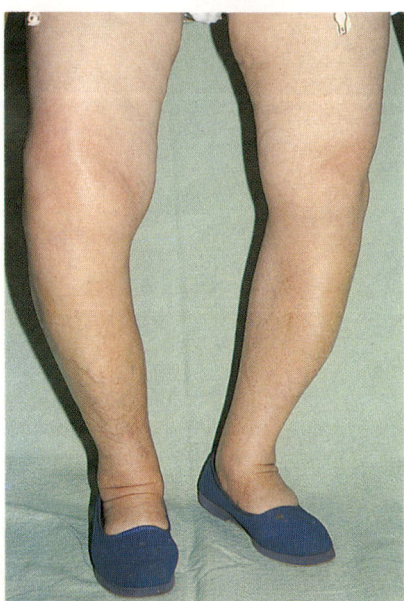

Fig.61 Paget's disease of the tibiae and fibulae. Thickening and softening of the bones has caused bowing of the legs.

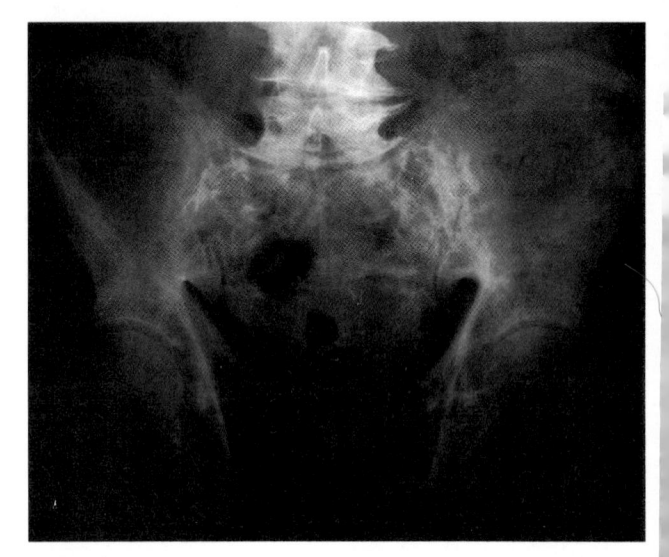

Fig.62 X-ray of the pelvis showing extensive Paget's disease. The characteristic radiological findings include lytic areas, thickening and sclerosis.

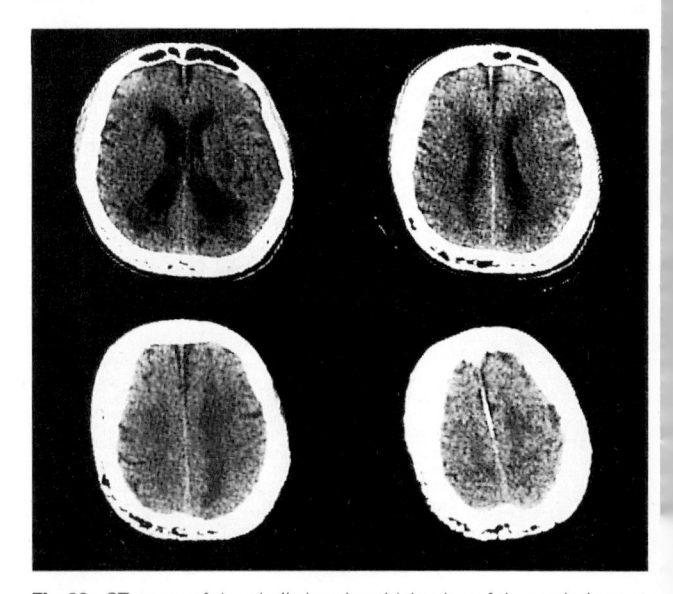

Fig.63 CT scans of the skull showing thickening of the vault due to Paget's disease.

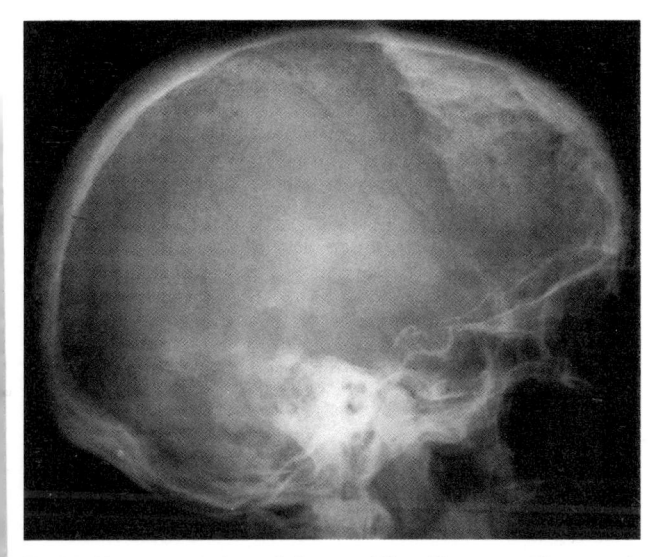

Fig.64 Hyperostosis frontalis interna. Wave-like areas of increased bone density are evident in the frontal region. This is a benign condition. The radiological appearance may be confused with Paget's disease or bony secondaries.

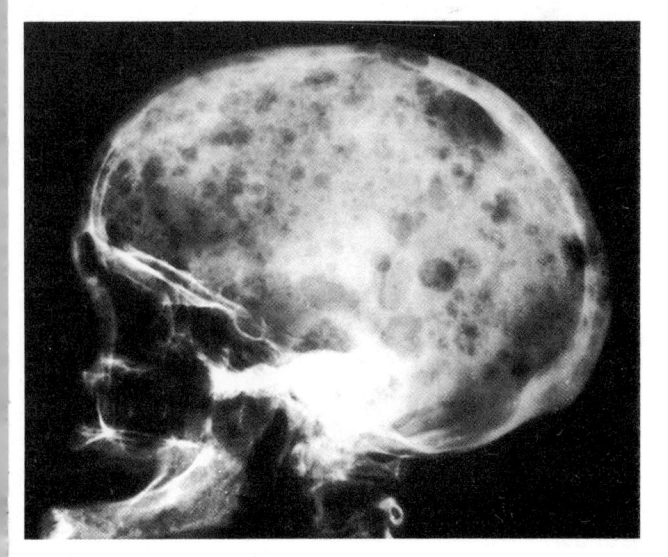

Fig.65 X-ray of the skull showing the classical appearance of multiple myeloma. Note the numerous 'punched-out' lytic areas.

Joint Disorders

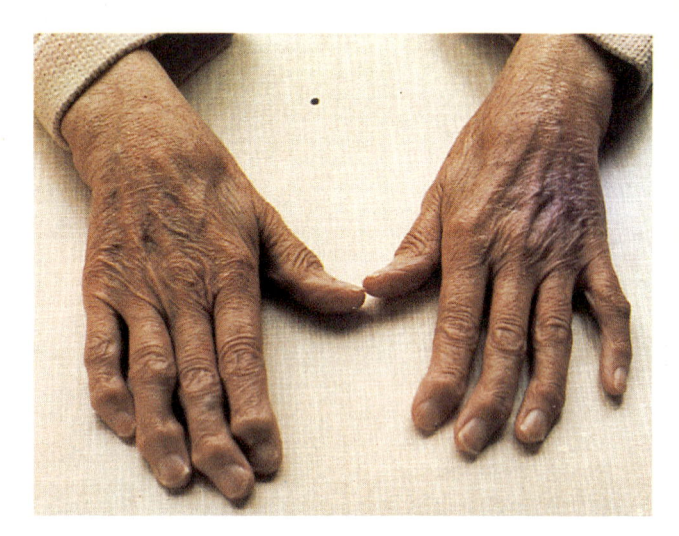

Fig.66 Osteoarthritis of the hands showing Heberden's nodes. These are bony swellings in the distal interphalangeal joints. Note the associated wasting of the small muscles of the hands.

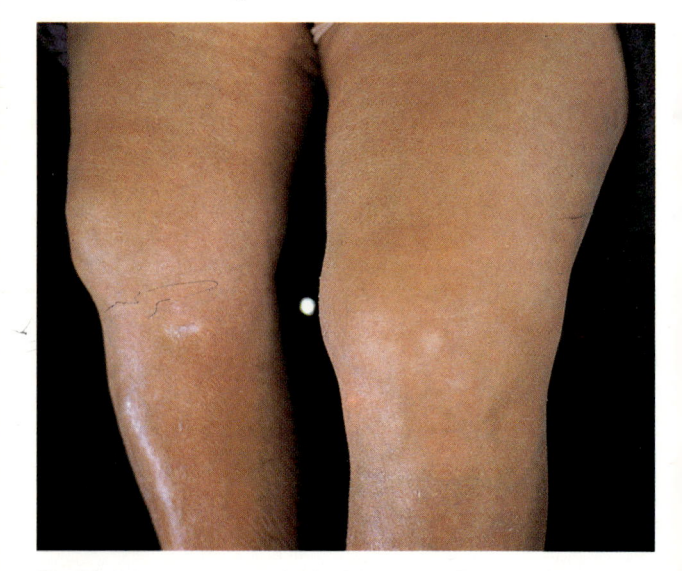

Fig.67 Advanced osteoarthritis of the knees. The symptoms include pain, swelling, deformity and difficulty in walking. Radiological investigation shows loss of joint space and sclerosis of the subchondral bone.

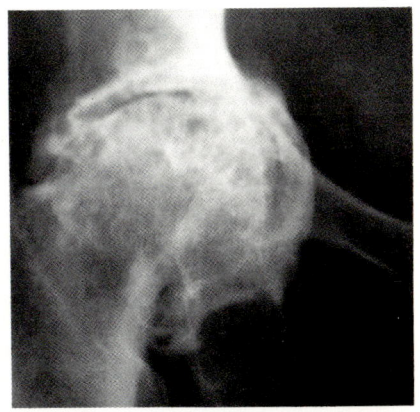

Fig.68 Advanced osteoarthritis of the hip joint showing complete loss of articular cartilage with small cystic areas in the head of the femur and subchondral bony sclerosis. Protrusio acetabuli is developing.

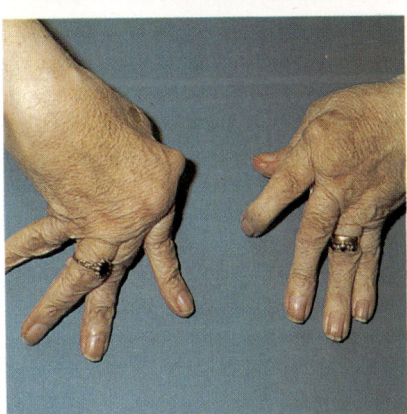

Fig.69 Rheumatoid arthritis involving the proximal interphalangeal, metacarpophalangeal and wrist joints (top). Hyperextension at the proximal interphalangeal joint caused by rheumatoid disease produces the classic 'swan-neck' deformity (bottom).

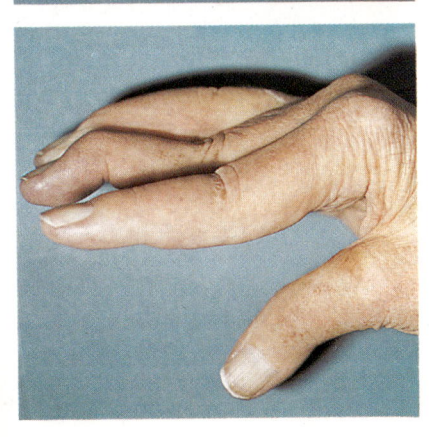

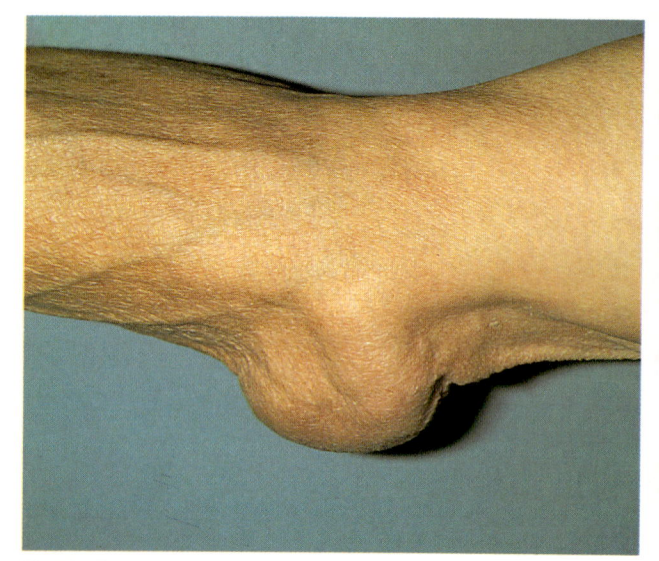

Fig.70 Rheumatoid nodule on the elbow. These are periarticular soft tissue swellings that occur around an area of vasculitis.

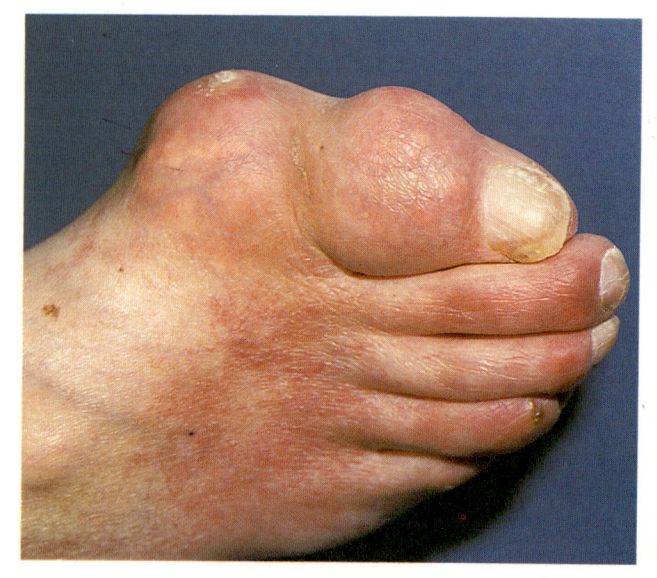

Fig.71 Gout is fairly common in old age. This elderly man presented with fever, vomiting and severe inflammation of the big toe.

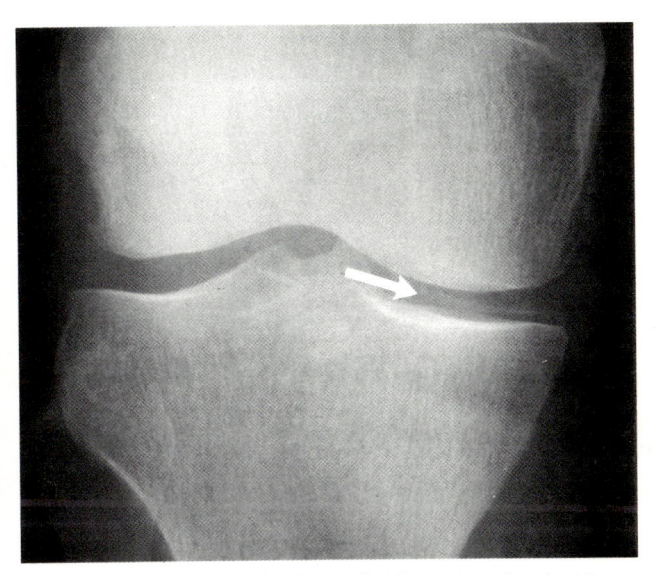

Fig.72 X-ray of the knee showing typical linear deposits of calcium pyrophosphate (arrowed) in a case of pseudogout.

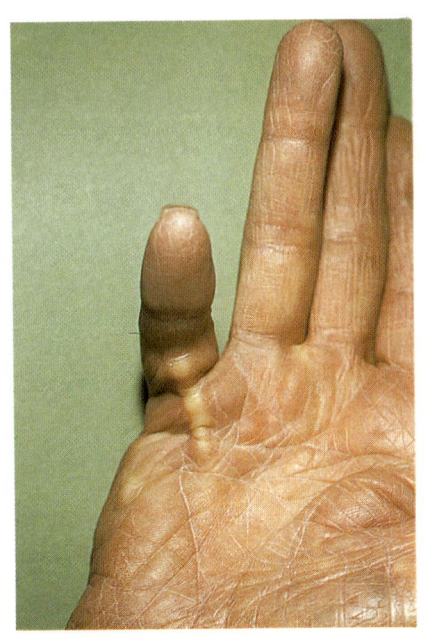

Fig.73 Dupytren's contracture is a common incidental finding in old people. It is a painless flexion contracture involving first the ring finger and then spreading to other fingers. It interferes with the fine movements of the hands and the patient may be unable to carry out the normal activities of daily living.

44

Cardiovascular Disorders

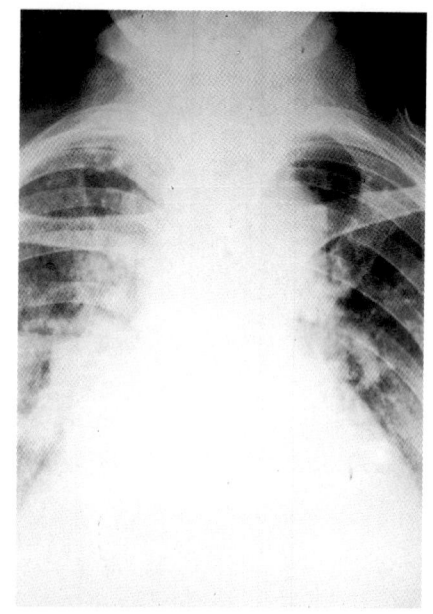

Fig.74 Chest X-ray showing cardiomegaly and pulmonary oedema in congestive heart failure, a frequent cause of emergency admission to geriatric wards.

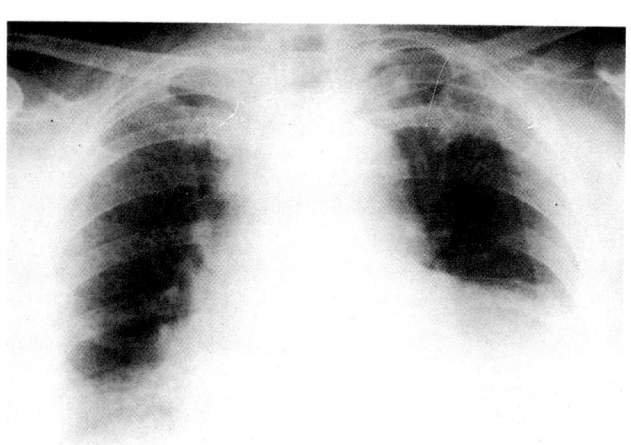

Fig.75 Left ventricular aneurysm due to previous myocardial infarction. This often leads to left ventricular failure and systemic embolism.

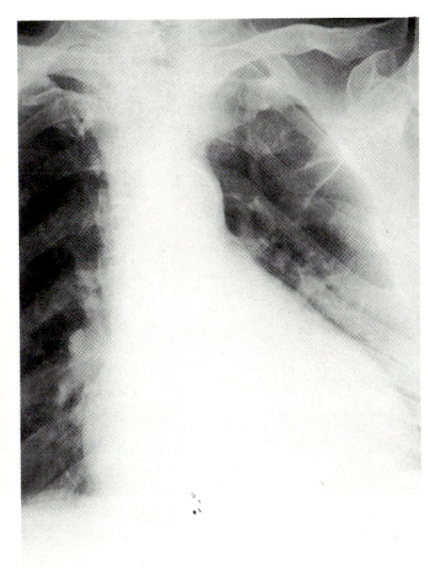

Fig.76 Left ventricular hypertrophy due to systemic hypertension. Good control of high blood pressure, even in old age, is worth achieving as it may reduce the risk of a stroke.

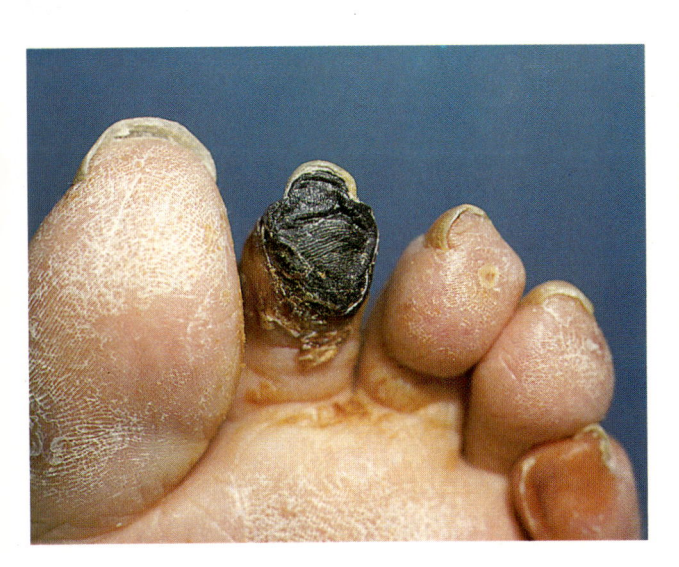

Fig.77 Embolic infarction of the toe due to subacute bacterial endocarditis. The underlying heart disease is now often aortic valve disease of uncertain aetiology rather than rheumatic mitral valve disease.

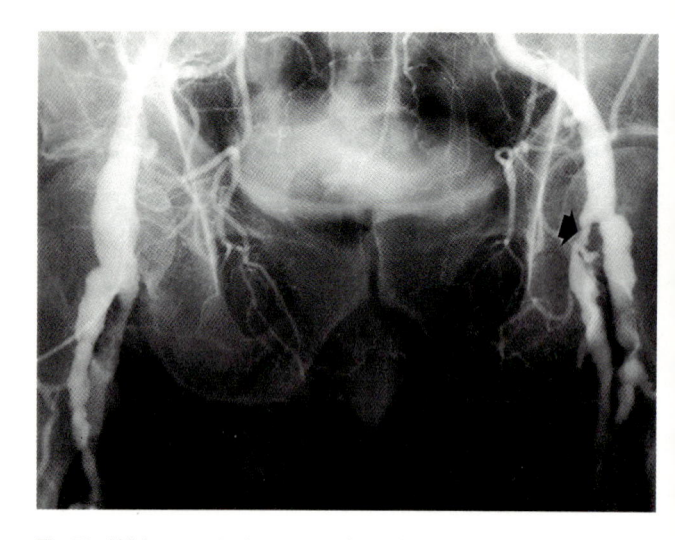

Fig.78 Widespread atheroma and arteriosclerotic narrowing (arrowed) of the large blood vessels to the lower limbs. Arteriosclerosis in the elderly gives rise to strokes, ischaemic heart disease, ischaemic colitis and peripheral vascular disease.

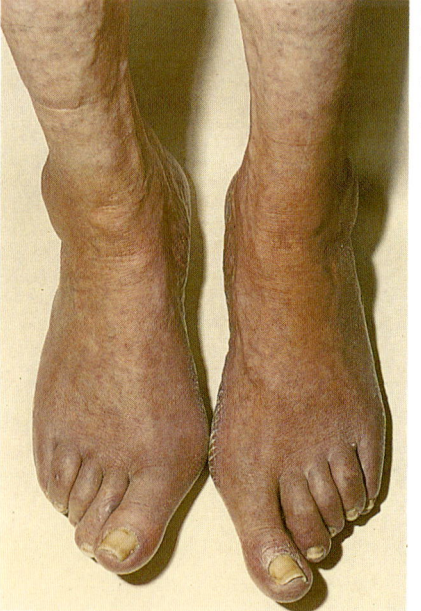

Fig.79 Peripheral vascular disease. The feet are painful, cold and blue and cause difficulty in walking.

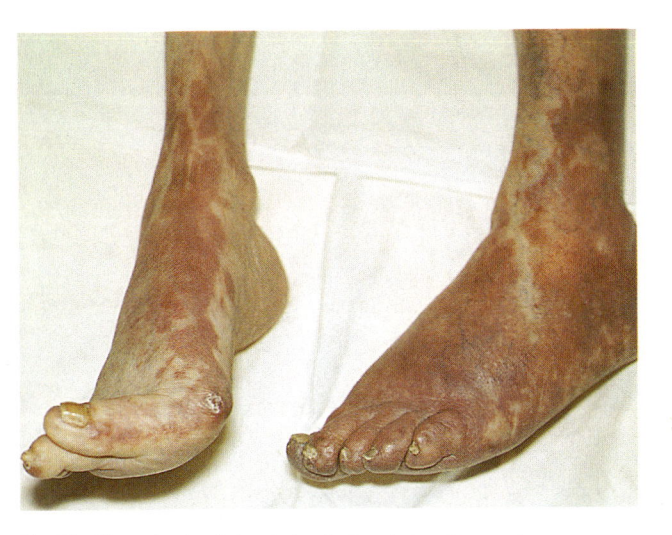

Fig.80 Thrombosis of the abdominal aorta is a frequent emergency in the elderly patient. Immediate vascular surgery may be life saving. This patient is developing ischaemic changes in the legs.

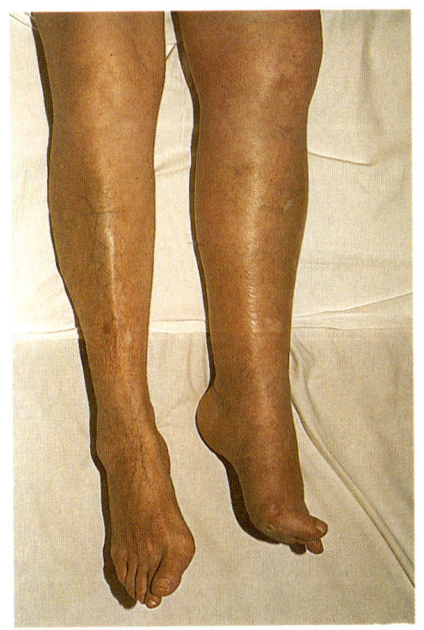

Fig.81 Deep venous thrombosis of the left leg due to immobility following an accidental fracture of the pelvis.

Disorders of the Chest

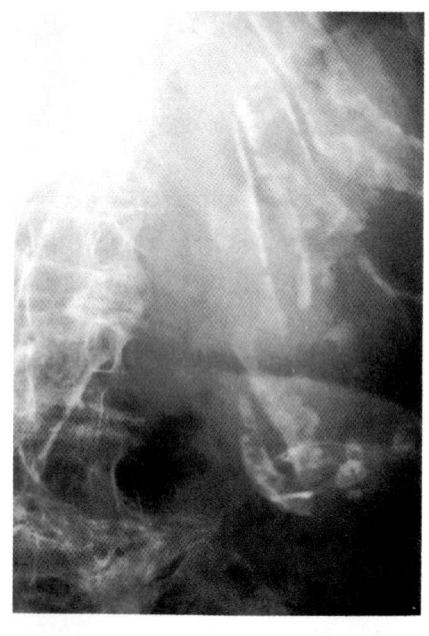

Fig.82 Calcified costal cartilages are almost universal in old age. This is a benign, age-related phenomenon and is sometimes confused with intrapulmonary or pleural calcification.

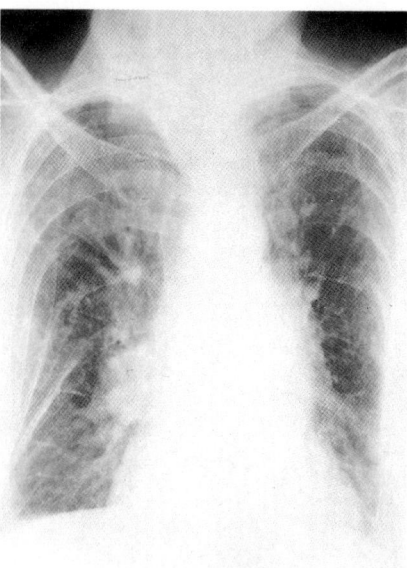

Fig.83 Typical radiological appearance of chronic bronchitis showing increased bronchopulmonary shadowing. Elderly patients may go on to develop cor pulmonale.

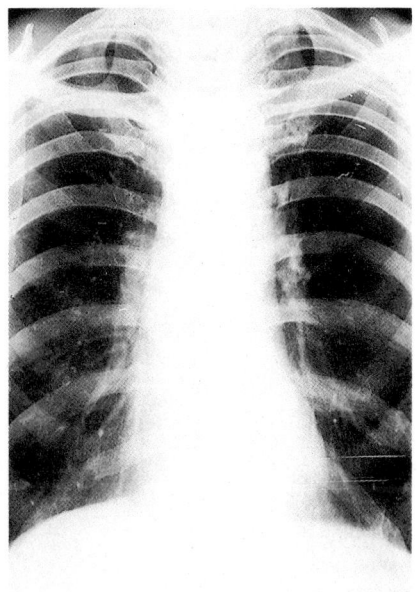

Fig.84 Chest X-ray of a case of emphysema showing increased translucency of the lung fields with a narrow cardiac shadow. The width of the intercostal spaces is also increased.

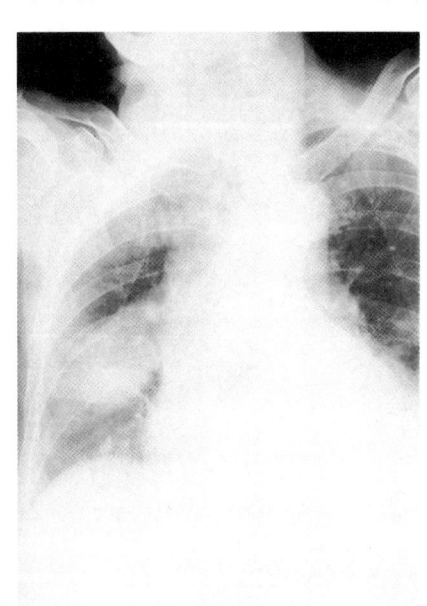

Fig.85 Right-sided basal infection secondary to carcinoma of the lung. In an elderly patient this is usually a terminal event.

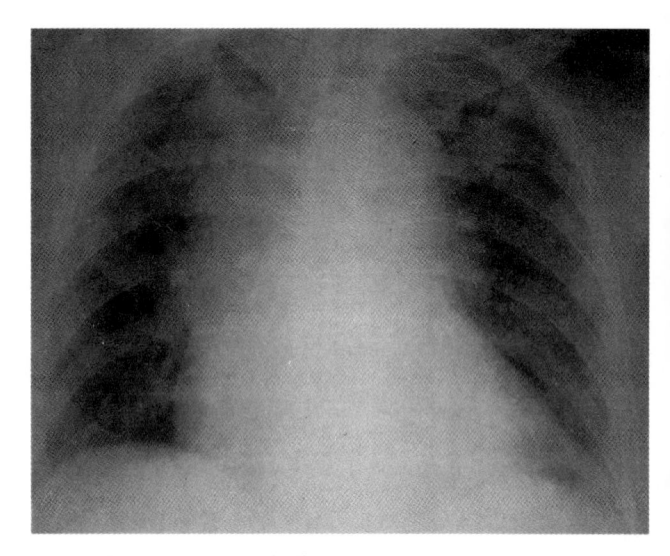

Fig.86 Bronchopneumonia. This is a frequent complication of various diseases of old age and carries a very high mortality. The response to antibiotic therapy is often poor.

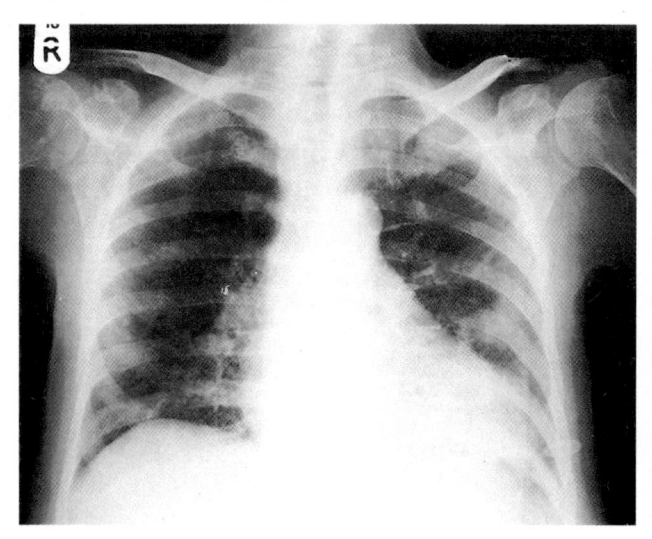

Fig.87 Chest X-ray showing fibrosing alveolitis associated with lupus erythematosis. The patient also had polyarthritis, anaemia, skin rash and a high erythrocyte sedimentation rate (ESR).

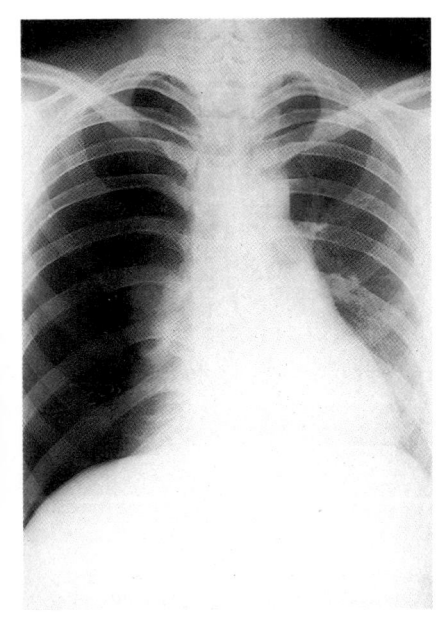

Fig.88 Chest X-ray showing a large, right-sided pneumothorax. In the elderly this condition can be painless and may present insidiously with dyspnoea, cyanosis and confusion.

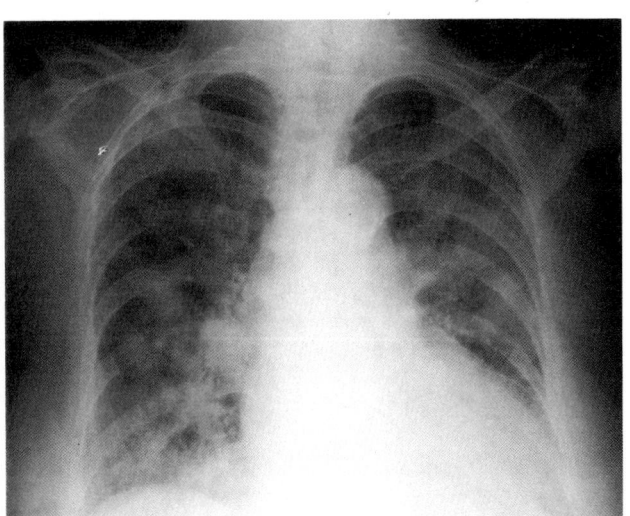

Fig.89 Round, discrete shadows of secondary deposits from carcinoma of the ovary. Tumours that tend to metastasize to the lungs are carcinoma of the breast and pancreas, hypernephroma, melanoma and carcinoma of the testicle.

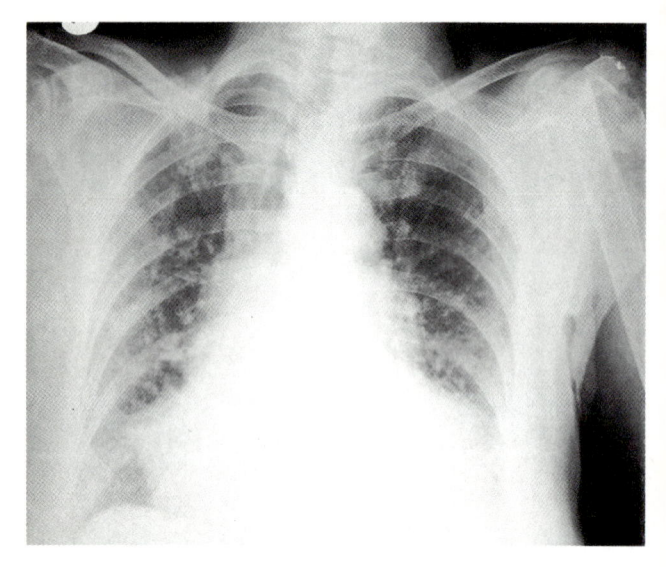

Fig.90 Miliary tuberculosis in a patient who presented with vague ill health. Occult tuberculosis is frequent in geriatric patients but very often the diagnosis is made too late as the clinical features are non-specific.

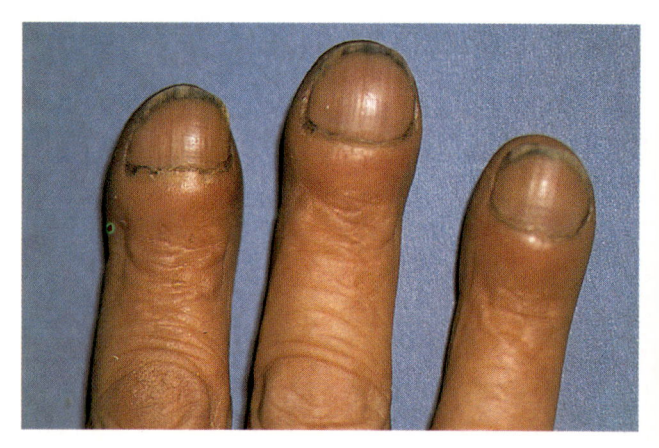

Fig.91 Finger clubbing. In elderly patients this condition is commonly due to carcinoma of the lung, chronic pulmonary infection, fibrosing alveolitis, bacterial endocarditis or cirrhosis of the liver.

Gastrointestinal Disorders

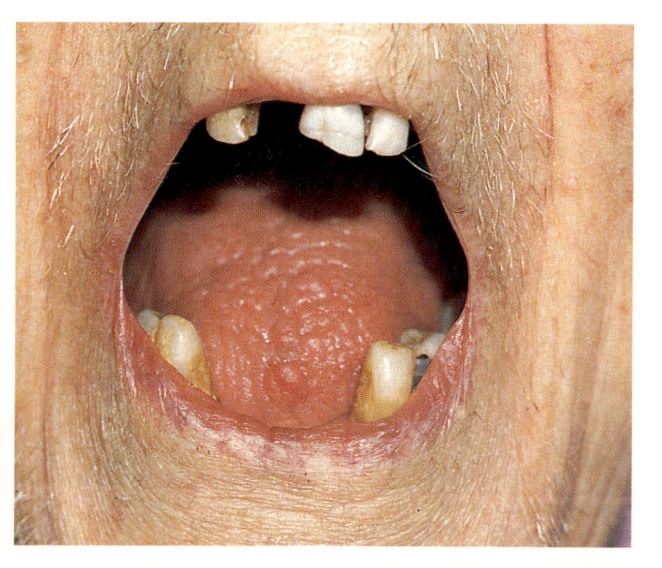

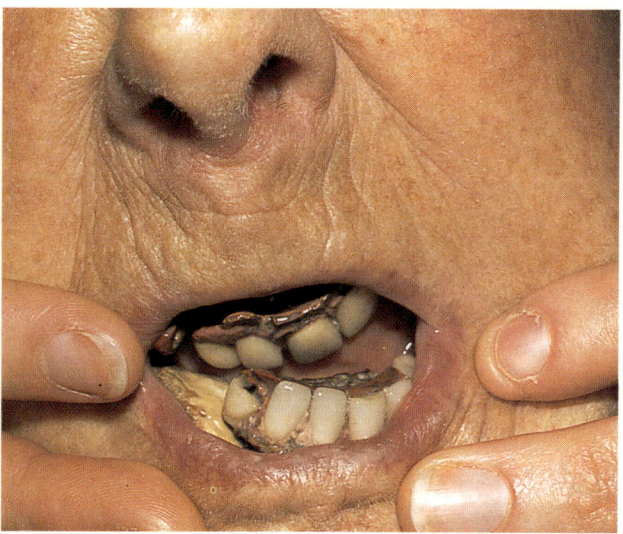

Fig.92 Poor oral hygiene is a frequent cause of malnutrition in the elderly. This patient (top) was unable to chew and presented with dehydration, weight loss and multiple vitamin deficiency. Old, ill-fitting dentures can also lead to poor nutrition in old patients (bottom). Dentures may fail to fit because of shrinkage of the gums and jaw with advancing age, stroke or facial palsy.

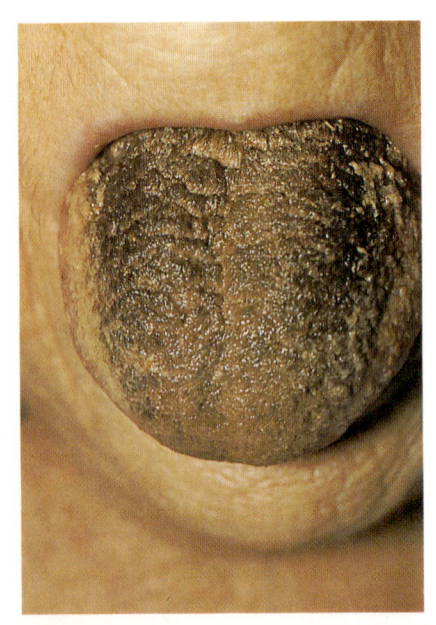

Fig.93 Severe dehydration causing extreme dryness of the tongue. The patient had fallen in her home and was discovered after two days, during which time she had been lying on the floor.

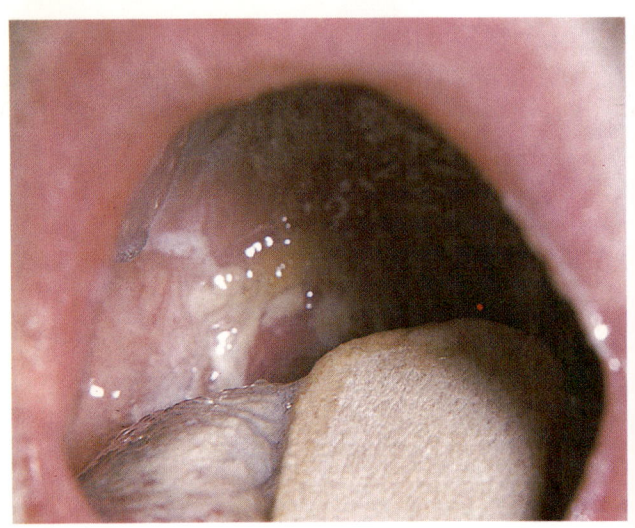

Fig.94 Candidiasis involving the oral cavity. The white patches of thrush are adherent and cause considerable pain and inflammation. Elderly patients frequently develop this condition during periods of ill health and debility.

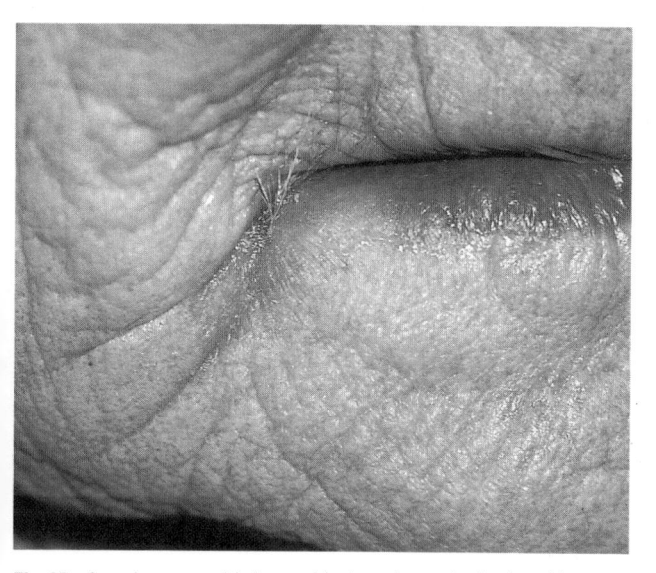

Fig.95 Angular stomatitis in an elderly patient who had multi-vitamin deficiency.

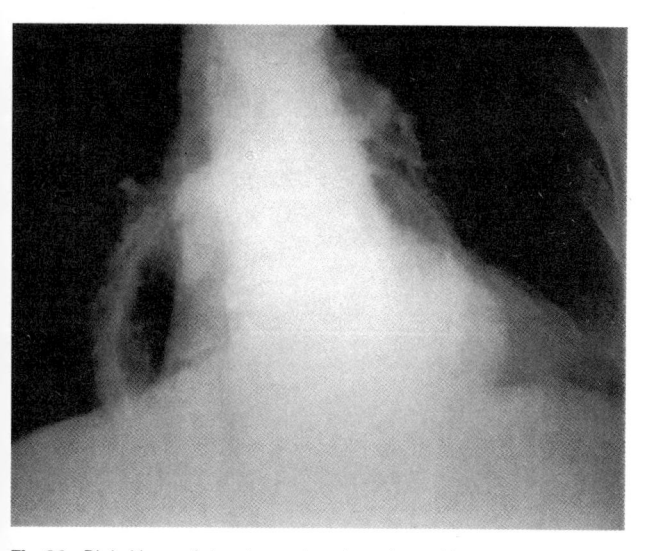

Fig.96 Plain X-ray of the chest showing a large hiatus hernia. Note the shadow containing an air bubble behind the heart. It is usually symptomless but may produce heartburn, dysphagia, retrosternal pain, chronic blood loss and anaemia.

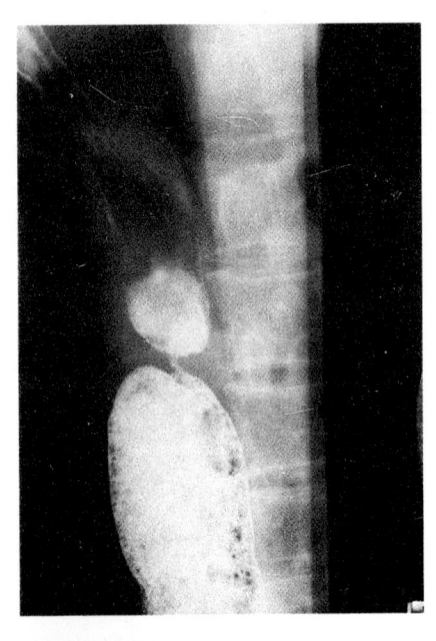

Fig.97 Barium meal X-ray showing oesophageal stricture due to long-standing reflux oesophagitis.

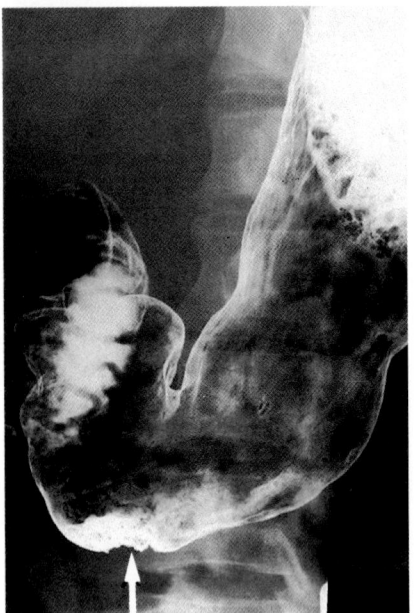

Fig.98 Barium meal X-ray of the stomach showing irregularity of the greater curve (arrowed). Endoscopy revealed a gastric carcinoma.

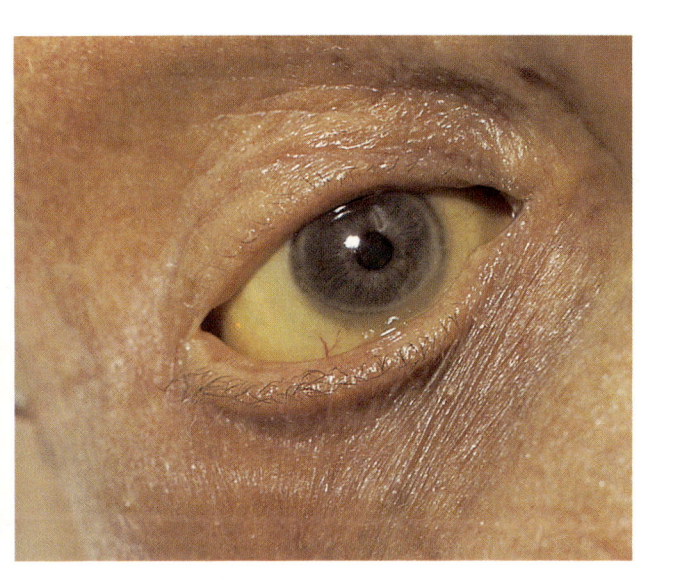

Fig.99 Jaundice due to carcinoma of the pancreas. The patient presented with anorexia, diarrhoea, weight loss and abdominal pain.

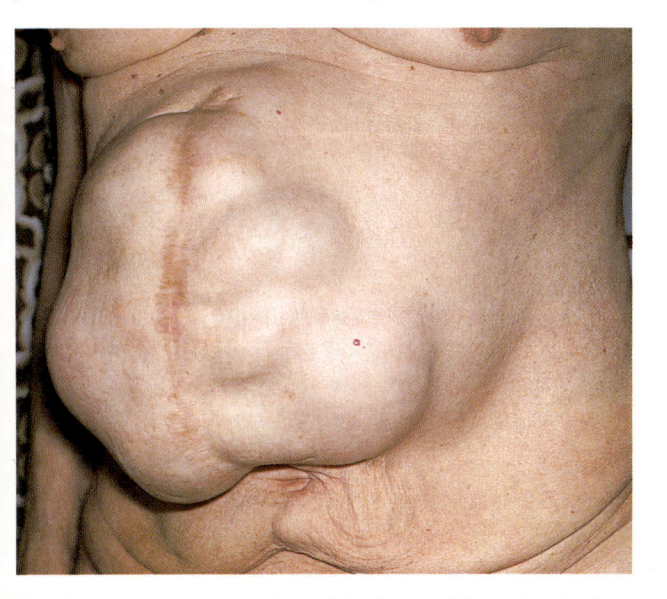

Fig.100 A large post-operative incisional hernia. The patient had absolutely no symptoms.

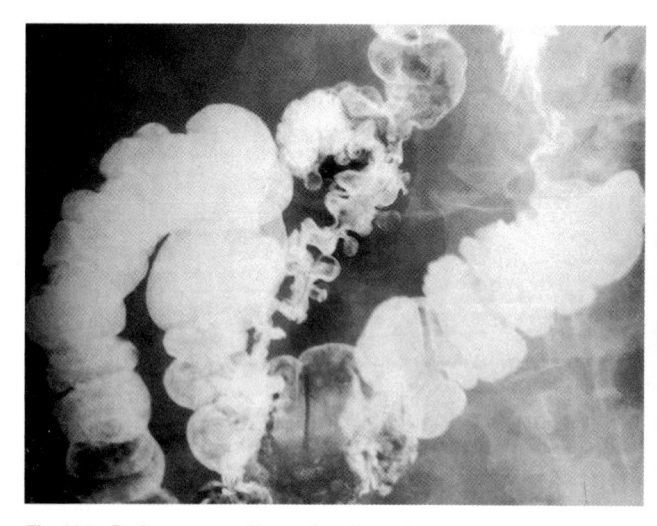

Fig.101 Barium enema X-ray showing colonic diverticulosis. This can be demonstrated in up to 50% of people over 80 years of age. It is usually asymptomatic but can cause pain in the left iliac fossa, constipation, diarrhoea, anaemia and anorexia.

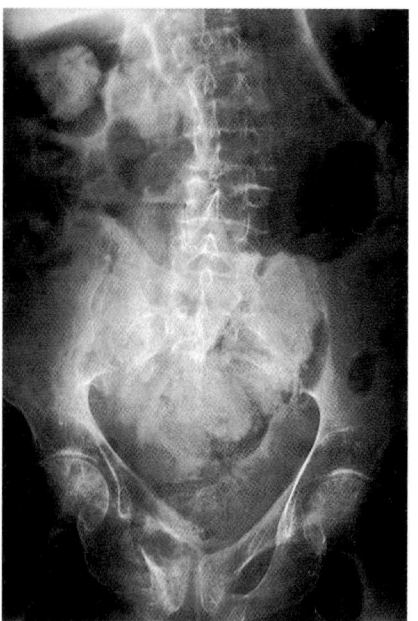

Fig.102 Plain X-ray of the abdomen showing the colon loaded with faeces. The patient had chronic constipation and presented with faecal impaction. Chronic and recurrent constipation is a common problem in old age.

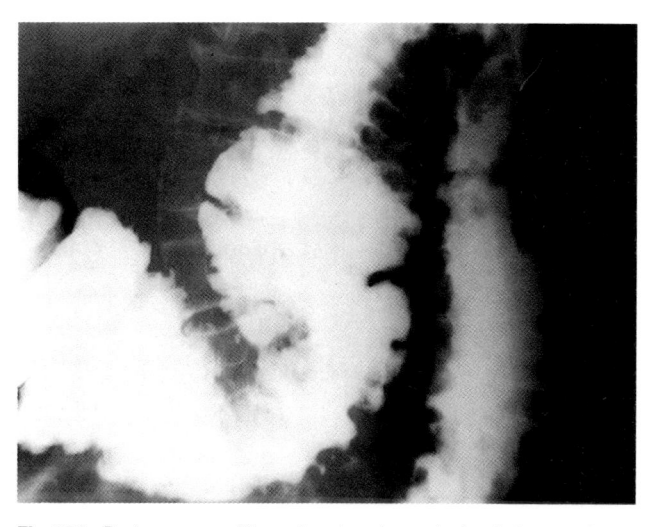

Fig.103 Barium enema X-ray showing the typical radiological features of ischaemic colitis. Note the 'saw-tooth' and 'thumb-printing' signs.

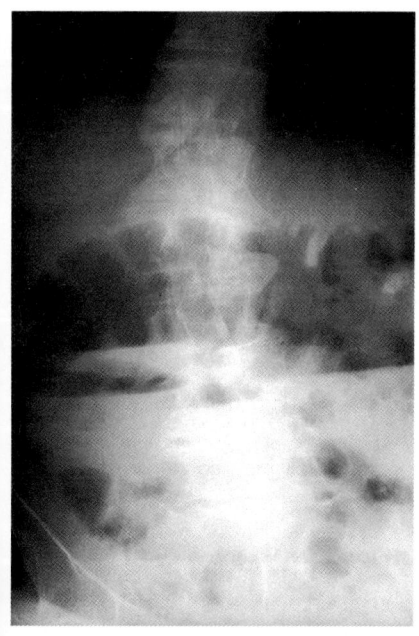

Fig.104 Plain X-ray of the abdomen showing multiple fluid levels in a case of intestinal obstruction. The patient had considerable abdominal distention but very little pain.

Muscular Disorders

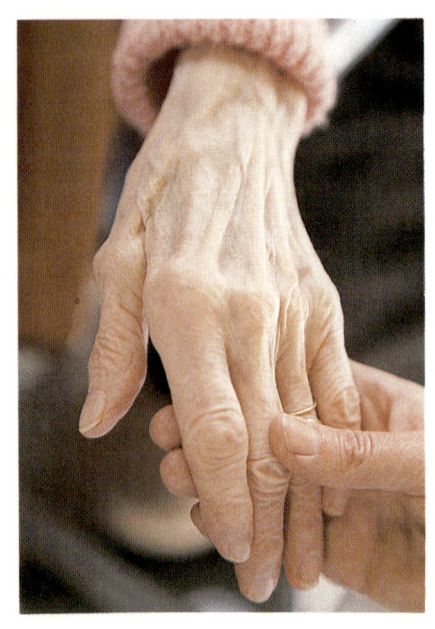

Fig.105 Wasting of the small muscles of the hand caused by a lesion involving the lower brachial plexus. Likely causes include cervical spine arthritis, scalenus anticus syndrome, Pancoast's tumour and vascular lesions.

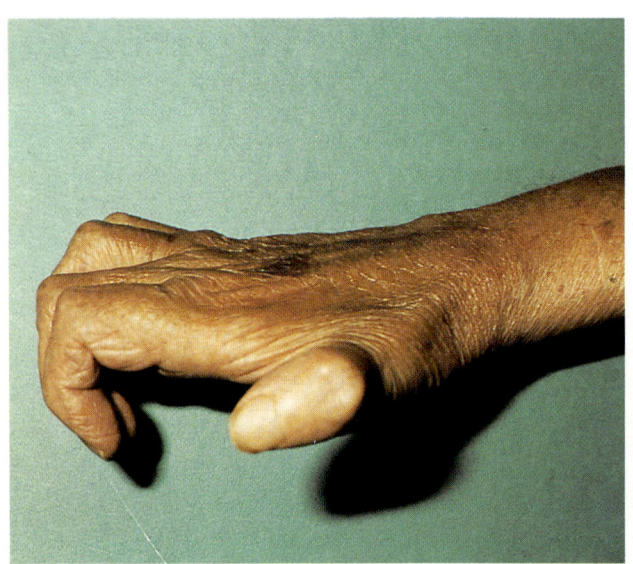

Fig.106 Claw-hand deformity with wasting of the small muscles due to an ulnar nerve palsy.

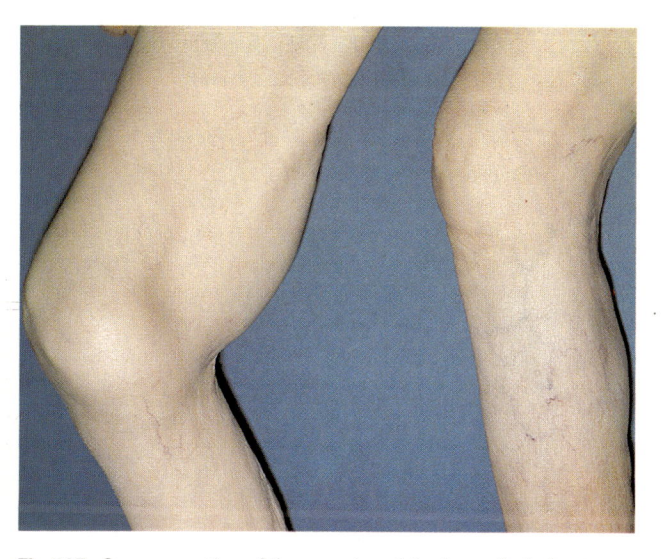

Fig.107 Severe wasting of the muscles of the lower limb due to chronic cerebrovascular disease. The patient may go on to develop contractures.

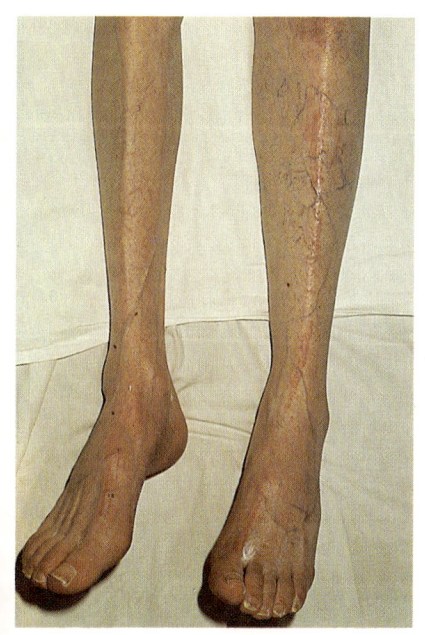

Fig.108 Wasting and paralysis of the legs due to motor neurone disease. This is due to degeneration of anterior horn cells in the spinal cord and in the motor cranial nuclei and pyramidal tracts. In the elderly the disease tends to run a chronic course.

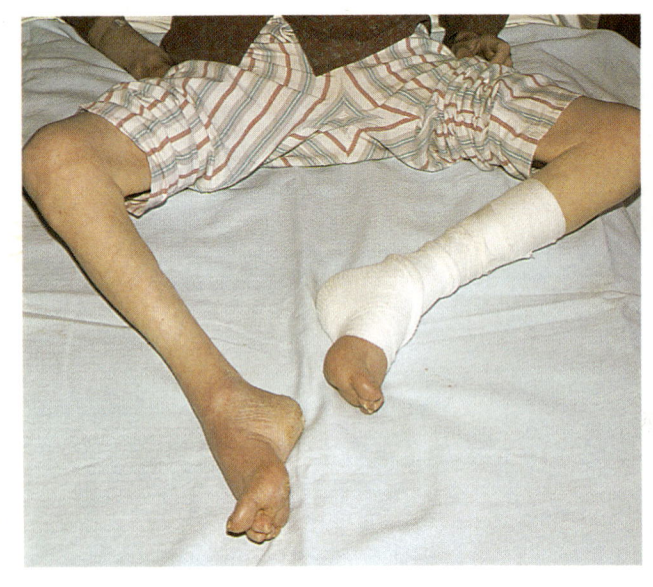

Fig.109 Spasticity of the leg muscles due to a spinal cord lesion.

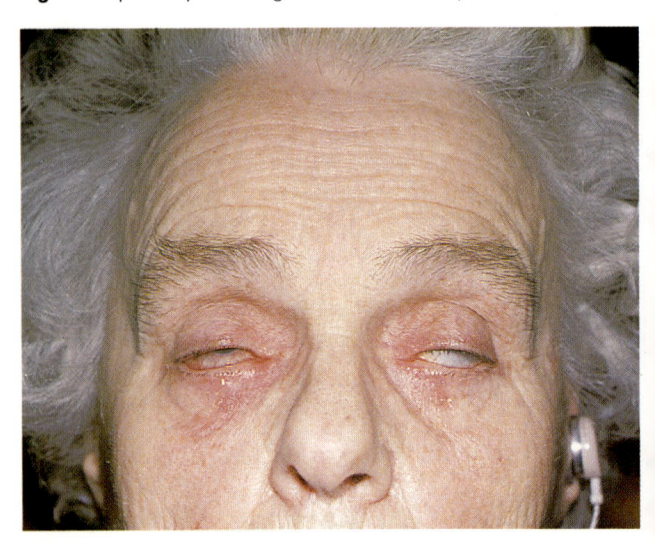

Fig.110 Myasthenia gravis. The face of an elderly lady showing bilateral ptosis and arching of the eyebrows. Such patients should be investigated for an occult carcinoma, for example of the lung or stomach.

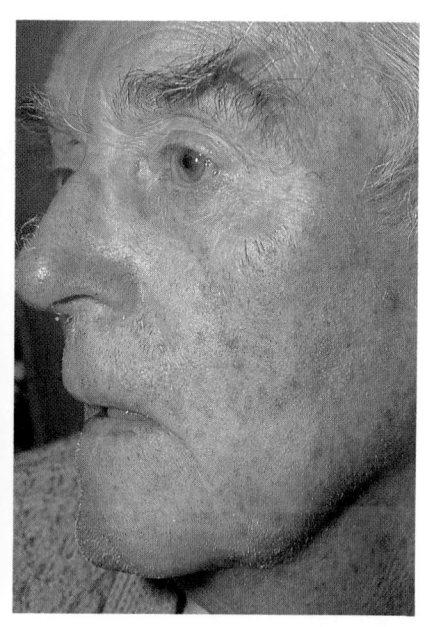

Fig.111 Facial rash and telangiectasia in a case of lupus erythematosus. The patient had general muscular weakness (polymyositis) with renal damage and cerebrovascular disease.

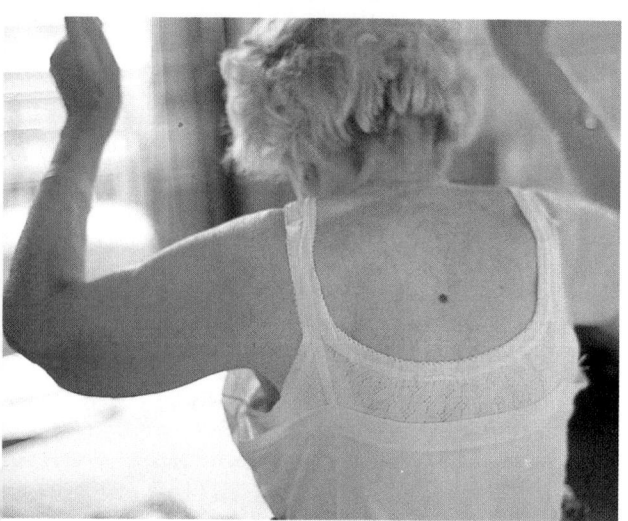

Fig.112 Polymyalgia rheumatica giving rise to pain, stiffness and weakness of the shoulder girdle muscles. The patient is unable to lift her arms above her shoulders. Many patients also have giant cell arteritis and the ESR is usually elevated.

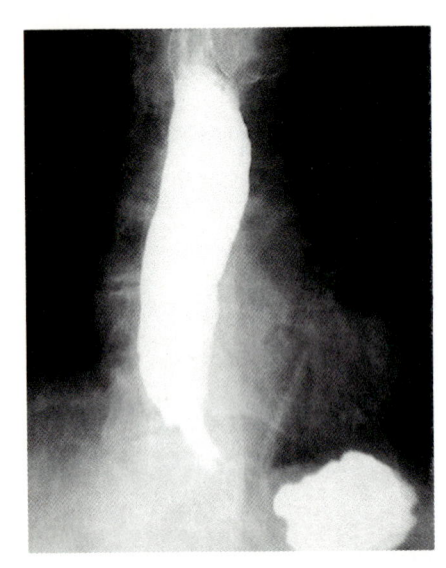

Fig.113 Barium meal X-ray showing oesophageal achalasia in a case of scleroderma. This elderly lady presented with dysphagia and malnutrition.

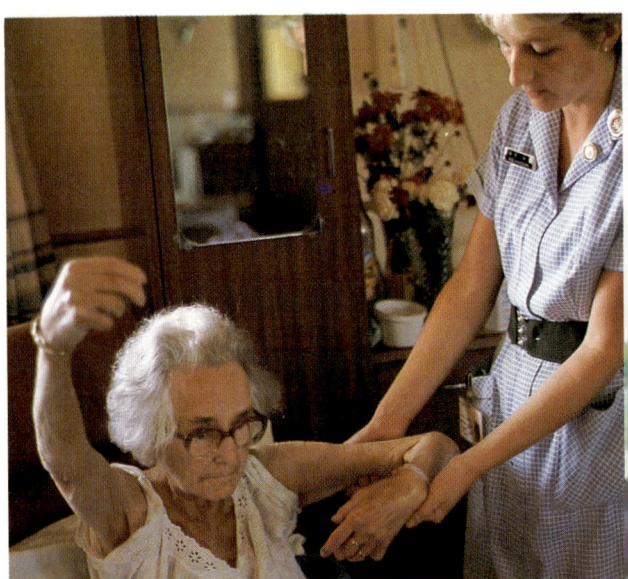

Fig.114 Frozen shoulder. The patient is unable to abduct the left arm at the shoulder joint, which is painful and stiff. This condition may be due to supraspinatus tendonitis or adhesive capsulitis, both of which are common complications of hemiplegia.

Skin Disorders

Only those skin conditions which are common in elderly patients are illustrated in this section.

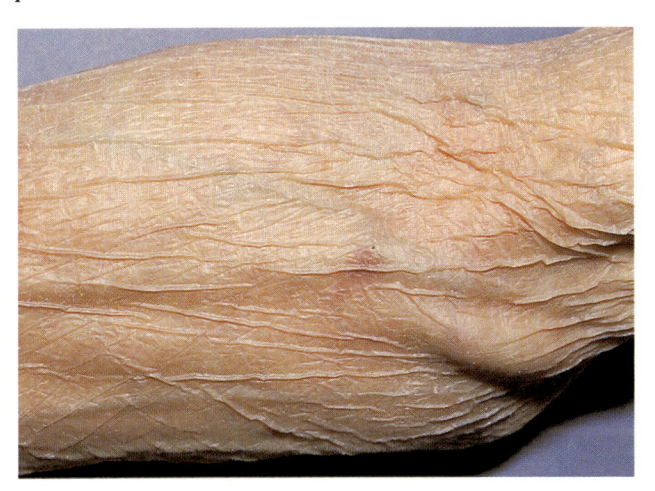

Fig.115 Senile atrophy gives rise to dry, tissue-like skin which is easily damaged. It is due to loss of collagen associated with advancing age. Connective tissue degeneration causes the majority of wrinkling of the skin associated with old age.

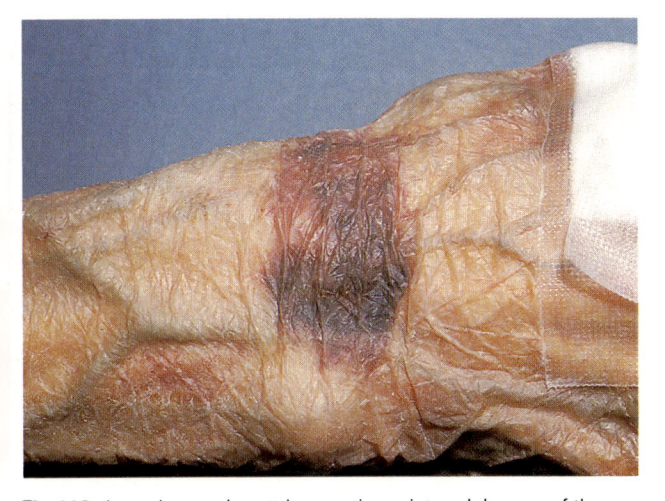

Fig.116 Irregular purple patches on the wrist and dorsum of the hand are typical of senile purpura. They are the result of increased capillary fragility, atrophic skin and trauma.

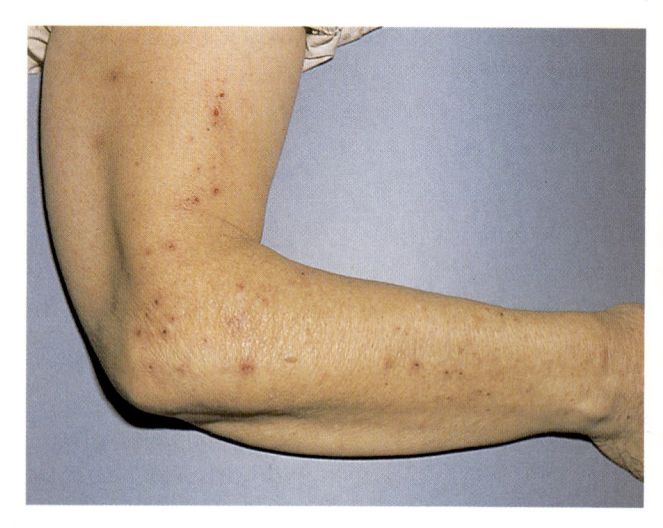

Fig.117 Pruritus is a common complaint in the elderly and scratch marks may be observed on the arms, legs and shoulders.

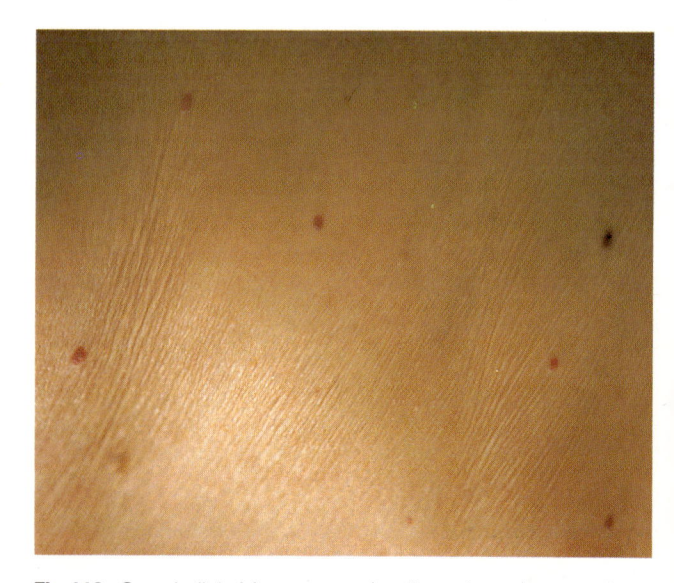

Fig.118 Campbell de Morgan spots (senile angiomas) are small benign, bright-red, raised spots on the skin of the trunk and shoulders. They are common in elderly men.

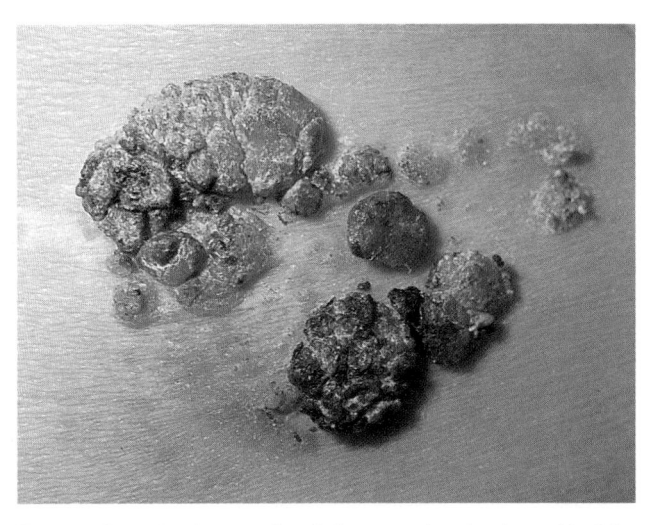

Fig.119 Seborrhoeic warts (senile keratoses) are benign epithelial proliferations that appear over the skin surface in old age. They are friable, warty, pigmented lesions and are often mistaken for malignant melanoma.

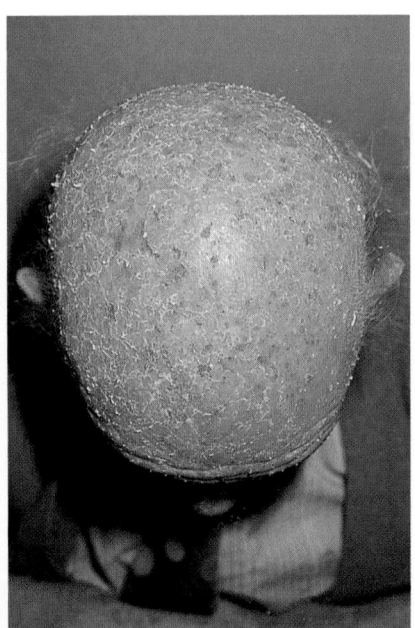

Fig.120 Ichthyoses are a group of disorders characterized by persistent and generalized scaling without any inflammatory change. The skin becomes dry with cracks in the stratum corneum and rhomboidal scales with flaky edges develop. Most ichthyoses are inherited but some cases occur with internal malignancy.

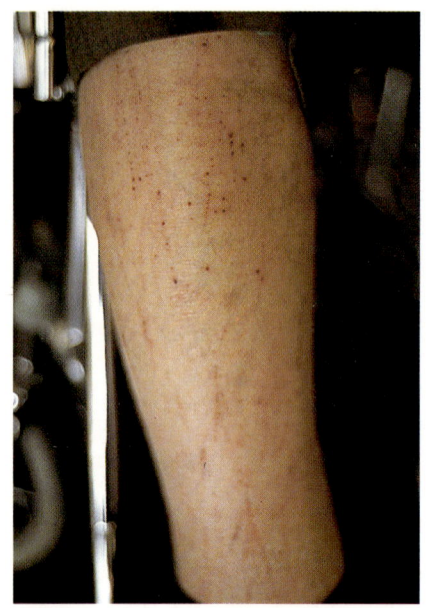

Fig.121 Scabies. Typical scratch marks of intense pruritus on the legs. This infestation occurs in elderly people who live in a state of self-neglect.

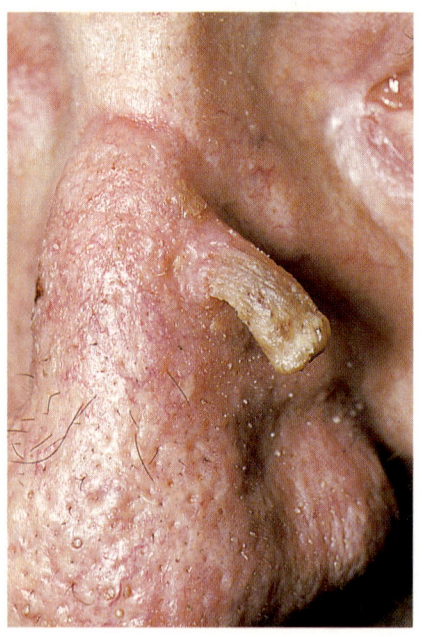

Fig.122 Squamous cell carcinoma arising as a 'horn' from the nose. This tumour appears in premalignant, sun-damaged skin and occasionally in chronic stasis ulcers.

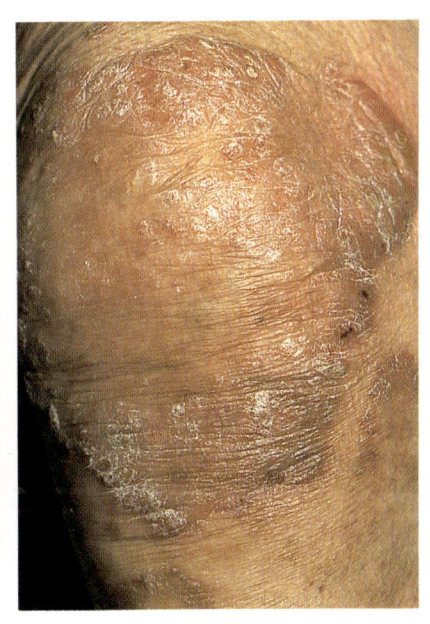

Fig.123 Psoriasis is seen frequently in elderly patients who may also have psoriatic arthropathy and typical nail changes.

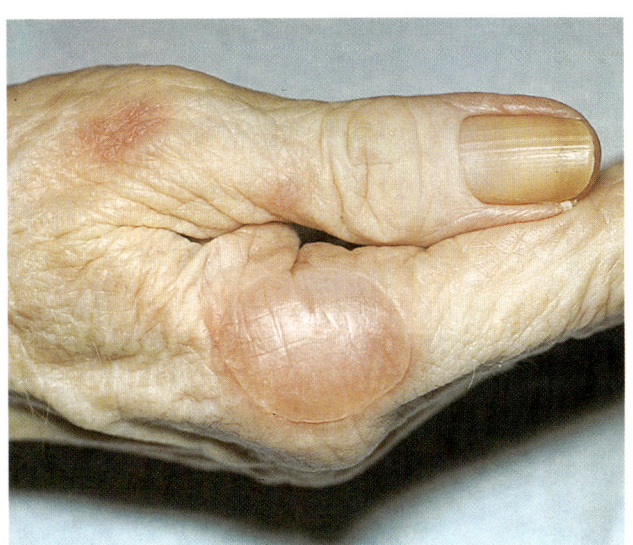

Fig.124 Tense bulla of pemphigoid. This is a skin disease of old age in which the blister forms below the epidermis, separating it from the dermis.

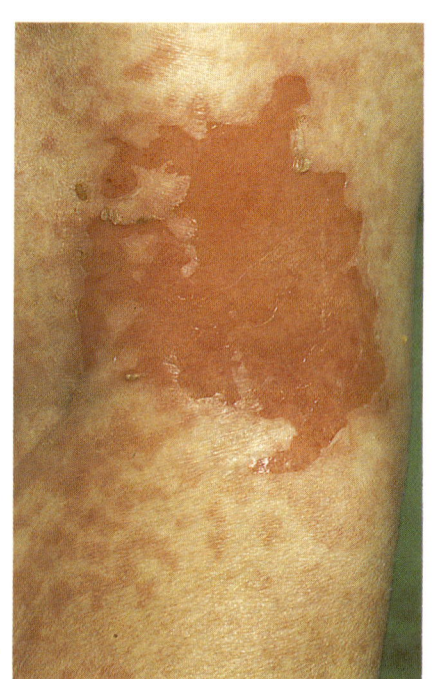

Fig.125 Pemphigus vulgaris is a more serious condition than pemphigoid. Here, the bullae are more fragile and the skin involvement is more extensive. The mucous membranes are frequently involved and the patient can be severely ill with pain, dehydration, secondary infection, toxaemia and confusion.

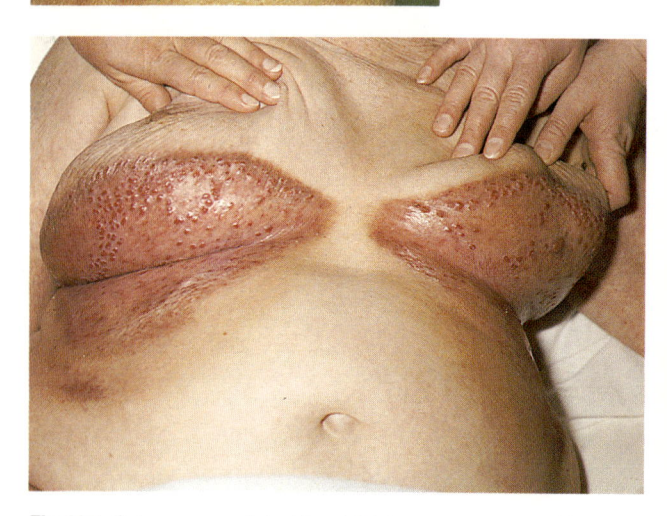

Fig.126 Submammary intertrigo. Moist, sore areas are evident under the breasts of this patient. This is a common problem in obese, elderly females.

Malignancy in Old Age

The presentation of malignancy in the elderly is very often atypical. The neoplasm may be found accidentally in a patient who is being investigated for an unrelated illness. Occasionally, the presenting clinical features are those of various non-metastatic complications such as myopathy, neuropathy, depression or dementia.

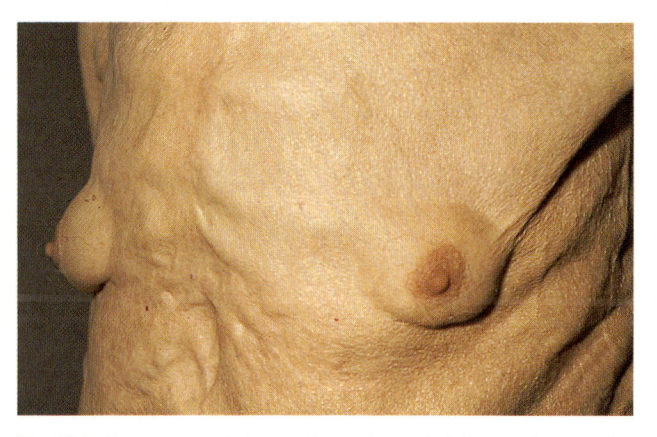

Fig.127 Gynaecomastia in a patient with underlying carcinoma of the stomach.

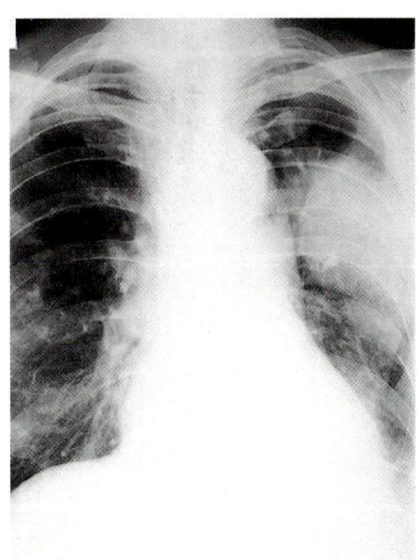

Fig.128 Chest X-ray showing left-sided bronchogenic carcinoma. This is a common malignancy in old age accounting for about one sixth of all deaths at age 65 and over.

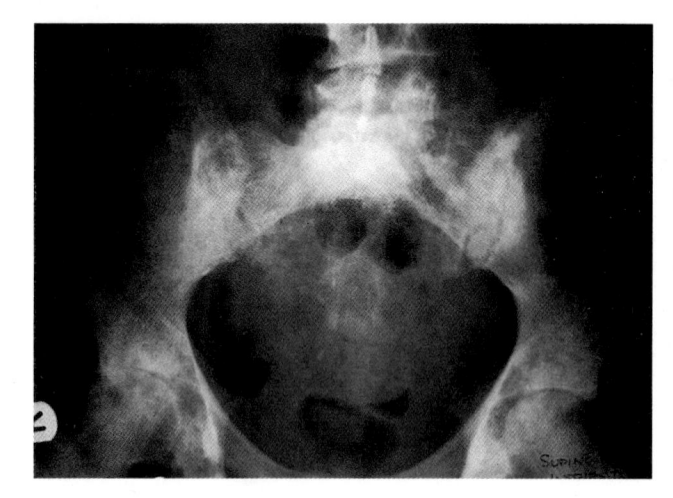

Fig.129 X-ray of the pelvis showing gross disorganization of the bony architecture due to secondary deposits from a carcinoma of the prostate. This is the most common malignancy in men over 65 years of age. It is often asymptomatic and discovered only on rectal examination.

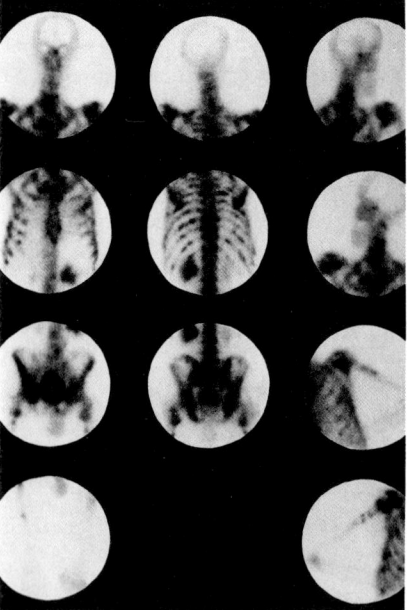

Fig.130 Isotope bone scan showing multiple 'hot-spots' due to bony metastasis from carcinoma of the prostate.

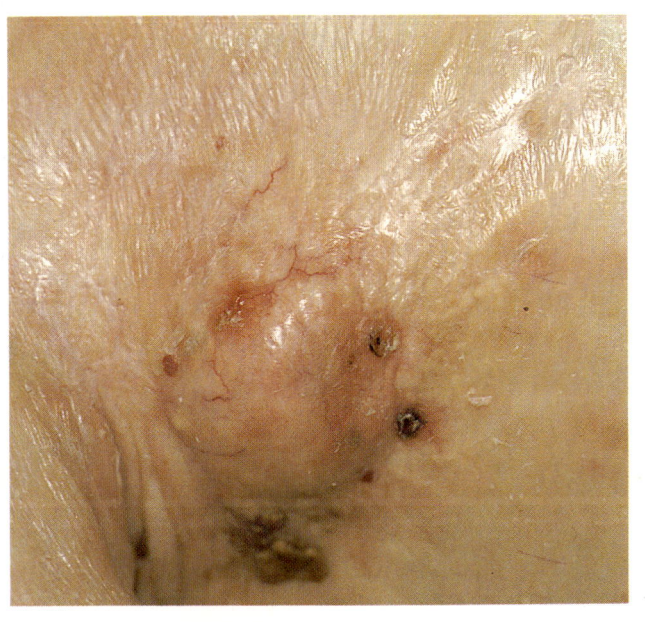

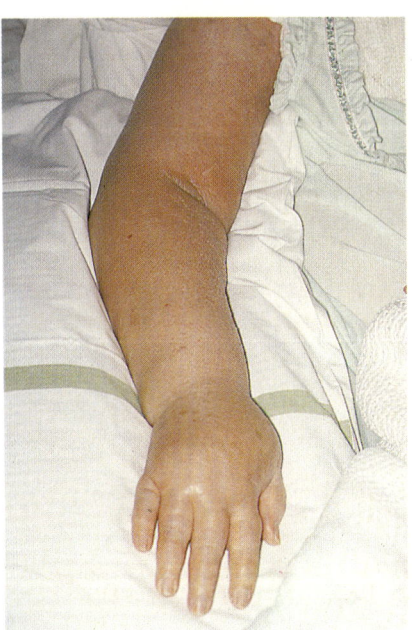

Fig.131 Carcinoma of the breast (top). This tends to run a chronic course in the elderly and some patients may simply ignore it. Brawny lymphoedema of the arm (bottom) may be an additional presenting feature.

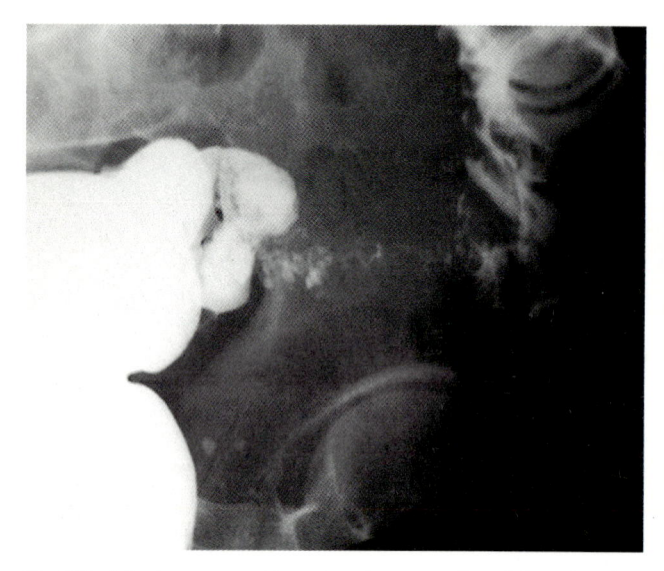

Fig.132 A barium enema X-ray showing narrowing of the colon due to carcinoma. This patient presented with a gradual change in bowel habit, malaise and weight loss.

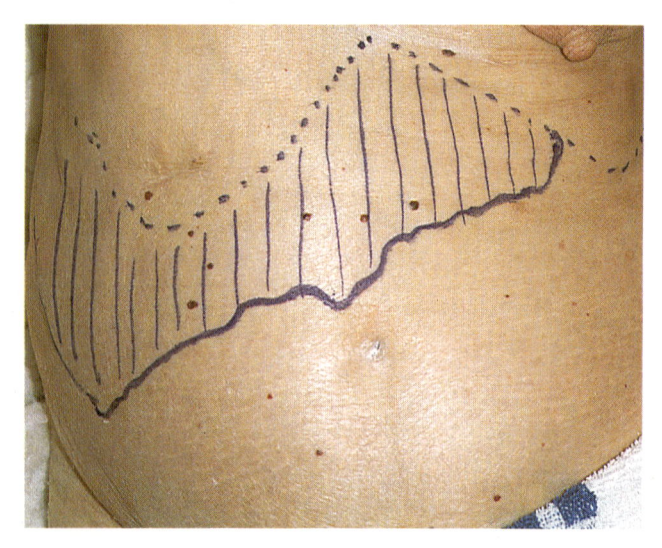

Fig.133 Gross hepatomegaly in an elderly lady due to metastases from an ovarian carcinoma.

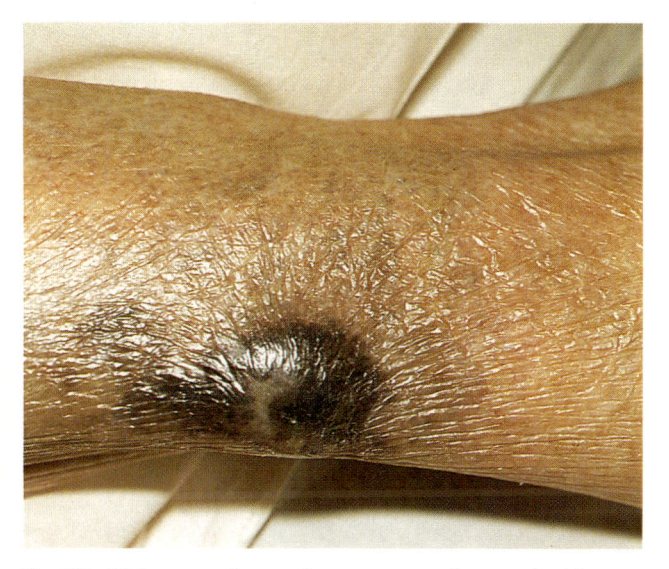

Fig. 134 Malignant melanoma is a common malignancy in old age. It arises from melanocytes and metastasizes early.

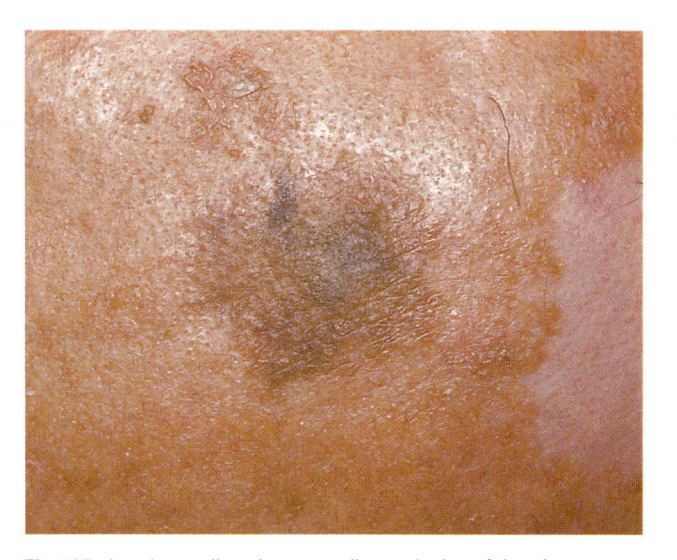

Fig. 135 Lentigo maligna is a premalignant lesion of the pigment cells. It occurs mostly on the face and spreads very slowly. Frequently, a malignant melanoma arises within the lesions.

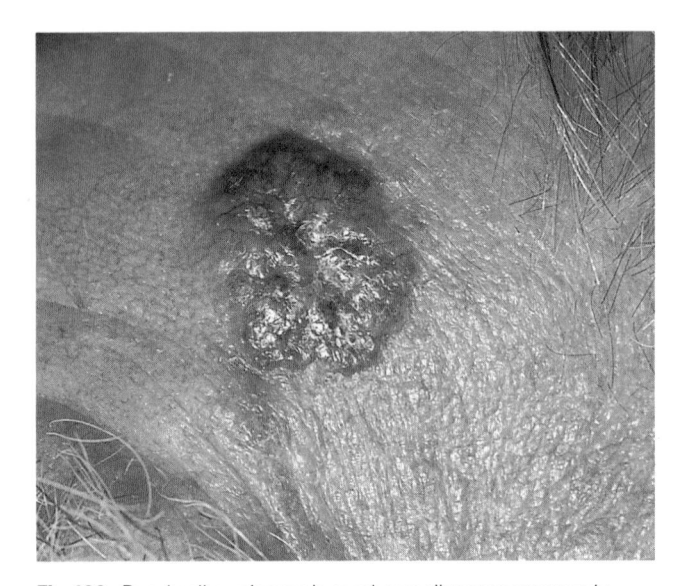

Fig.136 Basal cell carcinoma is another malignancy commonly found in elderly patients. It is usually found on the face, neck or ear, is slow growing and rarely metastasizes.

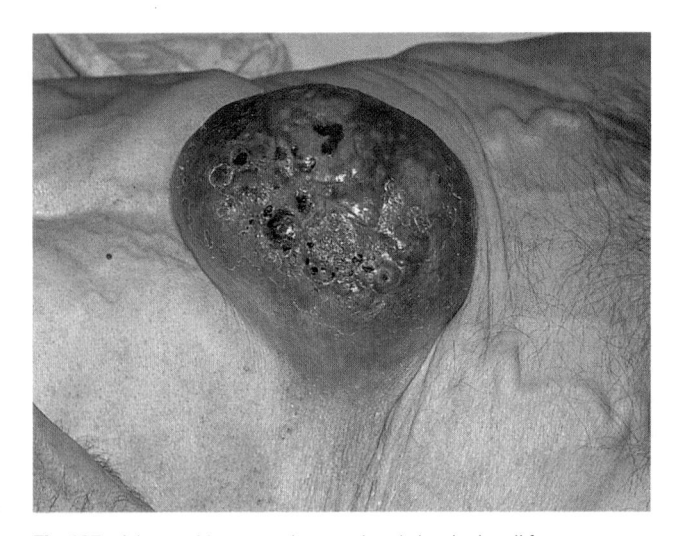

Fig.137 A large skin secondary on the abdominal wall from carcinoma of the bronchus. The patient had kept the lesion hidden for several months.

Miscellaneous Disorders

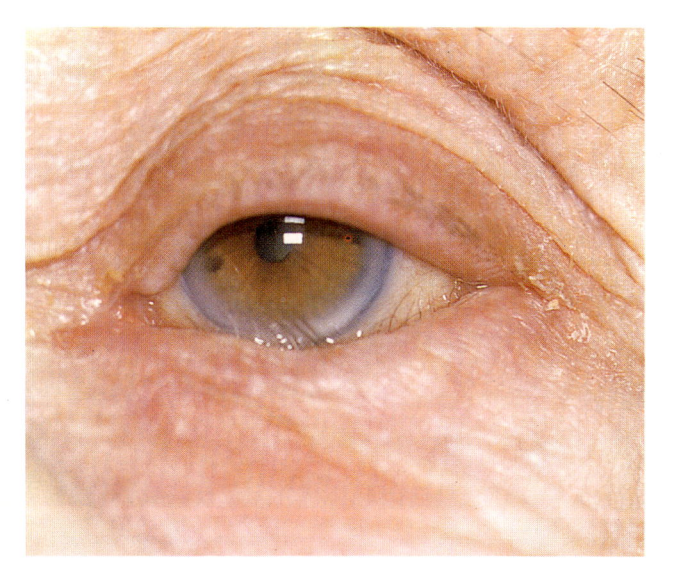

Fig.138 Arcus senilis is a common finding in the very old. It is formed by deposition of lipids at the periphery of the cornea. It should not be confused with Kayser-Fleischer ring or band keratopathy.

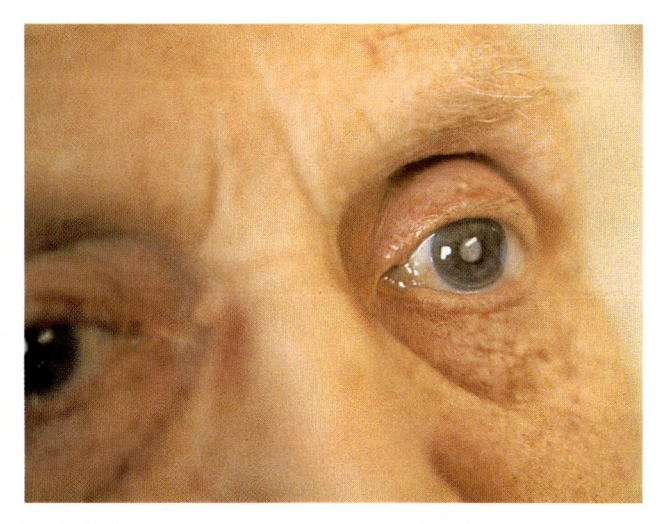

Fig.139 Cataracts are a frequent cause of visual impairment in the elderly. Ophthalmic surgery gives good results and can return patients to their previous independence.

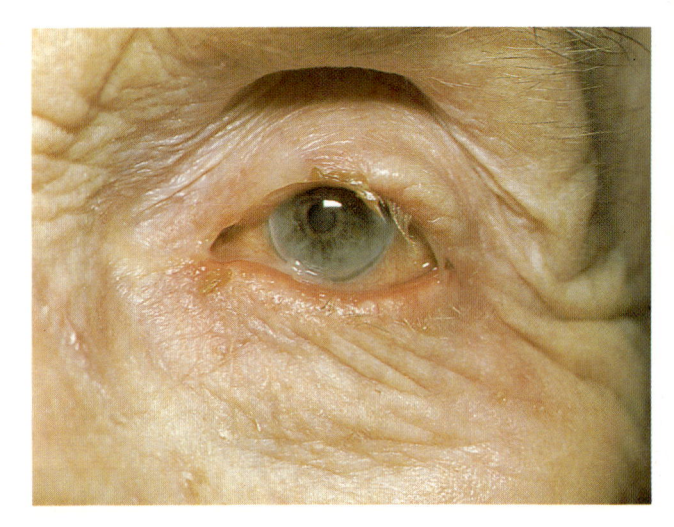

Fig.140 Conjunctivitis frequently occurs in elderly patients who are chronically ill. The aetiological agent is usually an adenovirus.

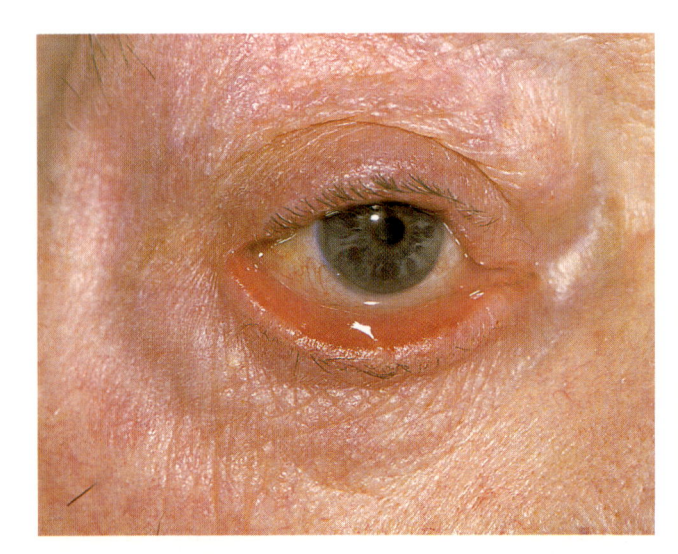

Fig.141 Chronic ectropion of the lower eyelid resulting in epiphora. Laxity of the eyelids in old age is an important aetiological factor.

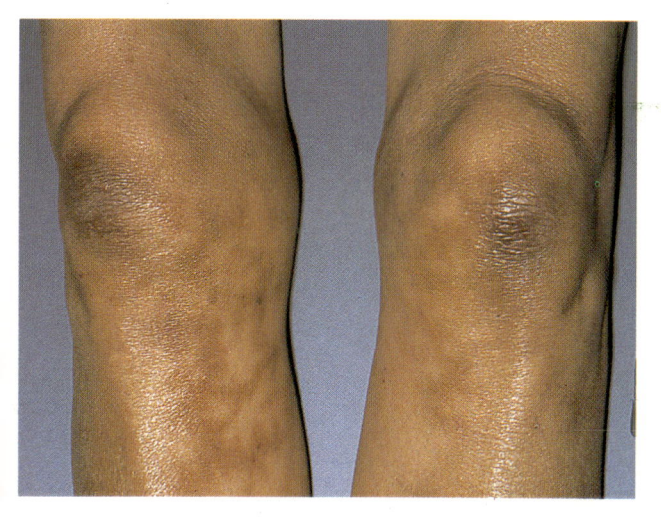

Fig.142 Erythema ab igne is seen in old people who live in cold houses and spend long periods in front of the fire. Such people are at risk from hypothermia and should be investigated for hypothyroidism.

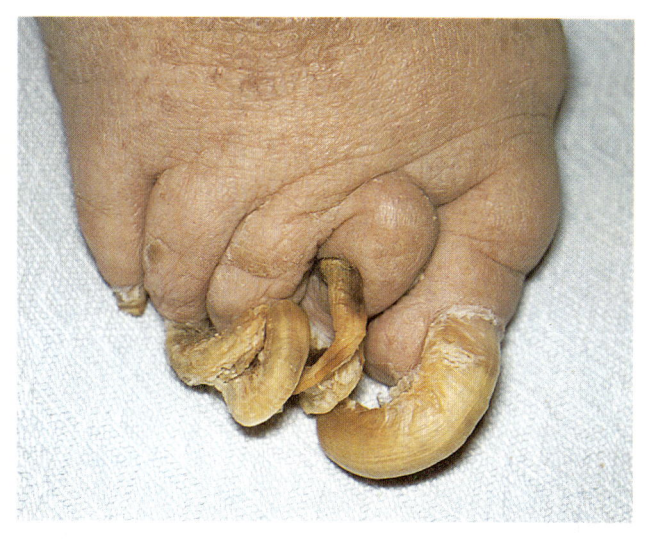

Fig.143 Onychogryphosis. Overgrown, claw-like toe nails are an important sign of social isolation and self-neglect. Such patients often suffer from depression, paranoid psychoses and dementia. They may present with falls or immobility.

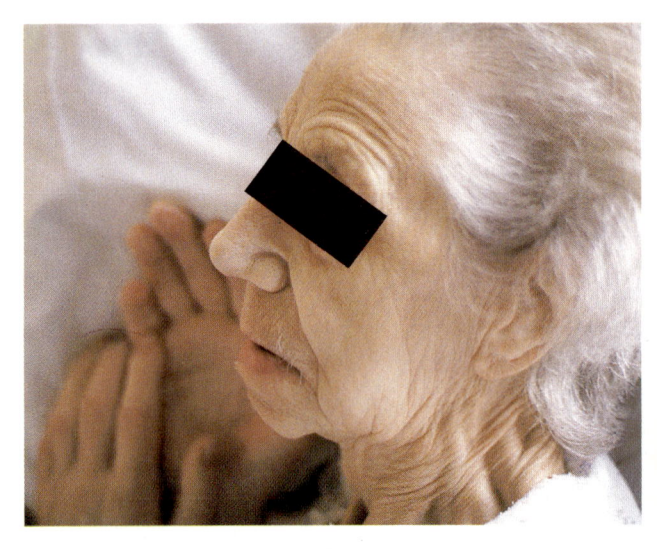

Fig.144 Hypochromic anaemia. Facial pallor due to severe anaemia, in this case secondary to chronic blood loss from a hiatus hernia.

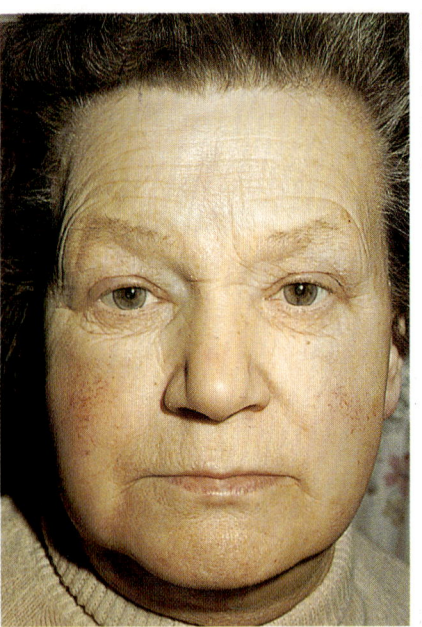

Fig.145 Pernicious anaemia. The face is typically pallid with a yellowish tint. Anaemias are found in 5-20% of the elderly population.

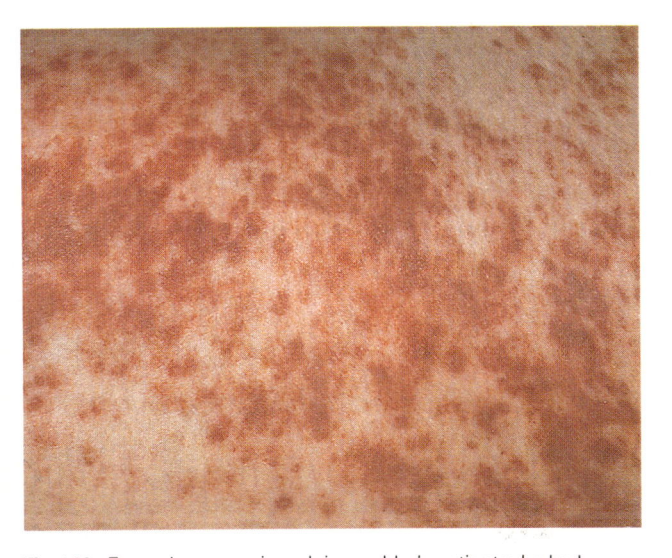

Fig.146 Extensive purpuric rash in an elderly patient who had developed thrombocytopenia secondary to treatment with methyldopa.

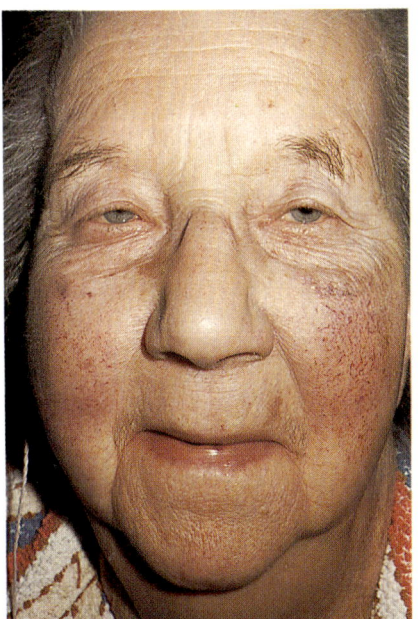

Fig.147 Hypothyroidism. The features are puffy and the skin coarse. The clinical features include physical and mental deterioration, constipation and increased sensitivity to cold. Myxoedema is common in the elderly, being found in 3-5% of admissions to geriatric units.

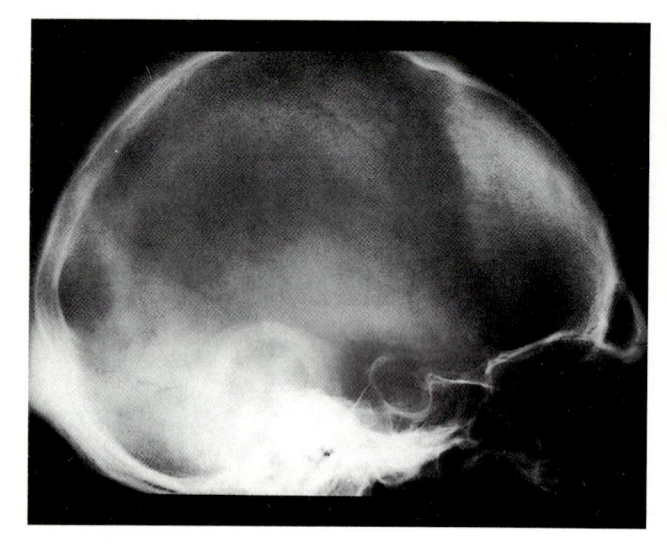

Fig.148 Acromegaly. This patient presented with weakness, hypertension and cardiac failure. X-ray of the skull showed enlargement of the pituitary fossa due to a tumour.

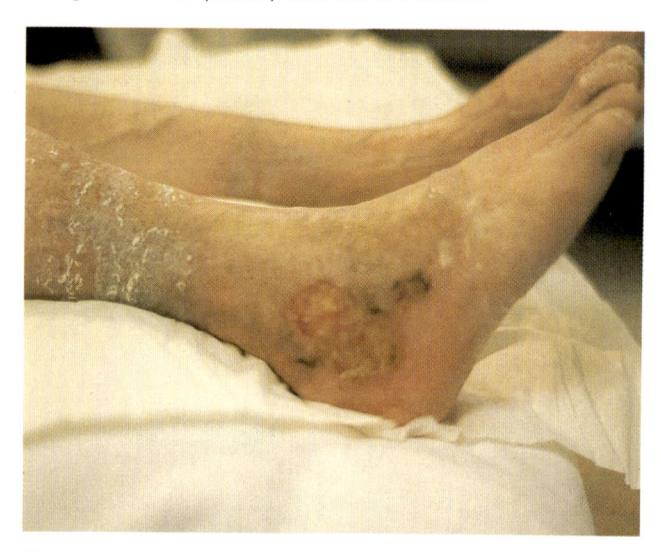

Fig.149 Diabetic ulcer on the lateral malleolus of an elderly patient. Such lesions occur in uncontrolled diabetes with small vessel disease. Maturity onset diabetes is frequent in the elderly population and usually responds well to treatment.

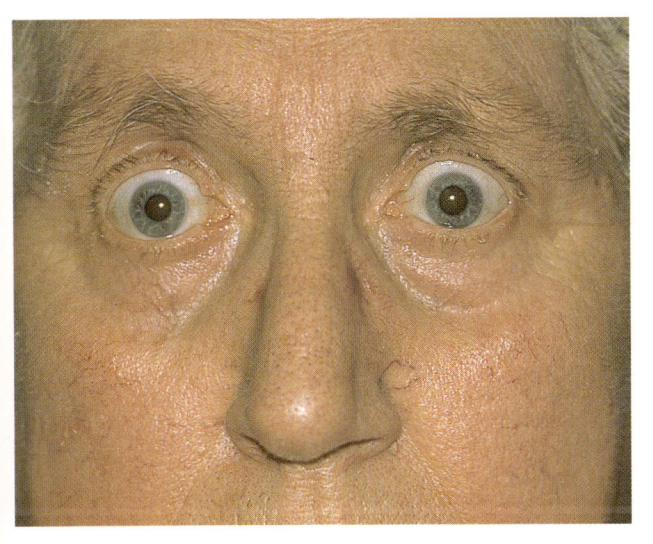

Fig.150 Thyrotoxicosis. Note the marked exophthalmos with lid retraction. This patient presented with depression, muscle weakness, diarrhoea and atrial fibrillation.

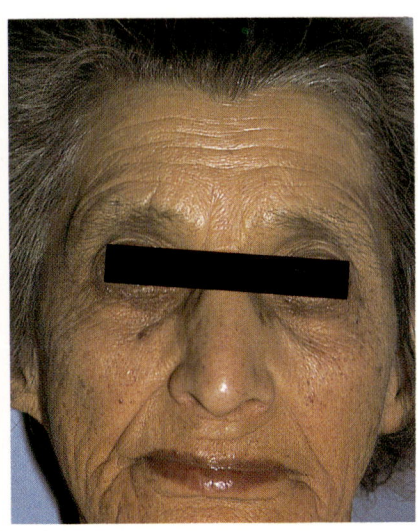

Fig.151 Facial appearance of a 75-year-old patient with Addison's disease. She presented with malaise, anorexia, hypotension and increased pigmentation,

Bibliography

Anderson, W.F. and Judge, I.G. (editors), *Geriatric Medicine*, Academic Press, 1974.

Brocklehurst, J.C. (editor), *Textbook of Geriatric Medicine and Gerontology*, 3rd edition, Churchill Livingstone, 1985.

Brocklehurst, J.C. and Hanley, T., *Geriatric Medicine for Students*, Churchill Livingstone, 1981.

Brocklehurst, J.C. and Kamal, A., *A Colour Atlas of Geriatric Medicine*, Wolfe Medical Publications Ltd., 1983.

Coni, N., Davison, W. and Webster, S., *Lecture Notes on Geriatrics*, Blackwell Scientific Publications, 1977.

Hamdy, R.C., *Geriatric Medicine, A Problem Solving Approach*, Ballière Tindall, 1984.

Maclennan, W.J., Shepherd, A.N. and Stevenson, I.H., *The Elderly (Treatment in Clinical Medicine)*, Springer-Verlag, 1984.

Pathy, M.S.J. (editor) *Principles and Practice of Geriatric Medicine*, John Wiley and Sons, 1985.

Rai, G.S. and Pearce, V. *Databook on Geriatrics*, MTP Press Ltd., 1980.

Index

Acromegaly, 83
Addison's disease, 84
Alveolitis, fibrosing, 51
Amaurosis fugax, 14
Anaemia
  hypochromic, 81
  pernicious, 81
Angiomas, senile, 67
Angular stomatitis, 56
Aorta, abdominal,
    thrombosis of, 48
Aortic arch, 12
Arcus senilis, 78
Arteriosclerosis, 47
Arthritis
  cervical spine, 5, 8
  osteoarthritis, 41-2
  rheumatoid, 42
Atheroma
  common sites, 12
  large blood vessels to
      lower limbs, 47
  vertebral arteries, 5, 8

Backward sway, 5, 9
Balance *see* falls
Bladder
  distension, 31
  filling defect, 31
  papilloma, 31
Bone
  disorders, 33-40
  metastatic carcinoma, 73
  see also fractures
Brain
  failure, 19-24
    classification, 19
  haematoma, 21, 22
  tumours, 15, 22

Breast
  carcinoma, 74
  gynaecomastia, 72
  submammary
      intertrigo, 71
Bronchi, carcinoma, 72, 77
Bronchitis, chronic, 49
Bronchopneumonia, 51
Bruising, 10

Calcification, costal
    cartilages, 49
Campbell de Morgan
    spots, 67
Candidiasis, oral, 55
Carcinoma
  basal cell, 77
  squamous cell, 69
Cardiomegaly, 45
Cardiovascular disorders,
    45-8
  falls and, 5, 6
Cataracts, 78
Cerebral infarction, 14-16
Chest
  disorders, 49-53
  infections, 50-1, 53
Circle of Willis, 12
Claw-hand, 61
Colitis, ischaemic, 60
Colon
  carcinoma, 75
  diverticulosis, 59
Confusion, 19-22
Conjunctivitis, 79
Constipation, 59
Cor pulmonale, 49
Corticosteroids and
    dementia, 20

Costal cartilages,
   calcification, 49

Dehydration, 55
Dementia, 19-24
   histological features, 23-4
   senile, 23
   steroid-induced, 20
Dentures, ill-fitting, 54
Diabetes, 83
Diverticulosis, 59
Drop attacks, 5, 8
Dupuytren's contracture,
   44

Elderly
   examination, 4
   hazards of minor
      illnesses, 4
   increase in numbers, 1, 2
   multidisciplinary
      treatment, 3
Emphysema, 50
Endocarditis, subacute
   bacterial, 46
Epiphora, 79
Erythema ab igne, 80
Exophthalmos, 84
Eye disorders, 16, 20, 78-9
Eyelids
   ectropion, 79
   ptosis, 16, 63

Faints, 5-10
   causes, 5, 6
Falls, 5-10
   causes, 5, 6
   complications, 5
Feet, oedema, 7

Femur
   fractures, 33-5
   pseudofracture, 37
Fibula
   bowing, 38
   fracture, 37
Finger clubbing, 53
Fractures
   femur, 33-5
   fibula, 37
   tibia, 37
   vertebral bodies, 37
   wrist, 10
Friction burns, 26

Gastrointestinal disorders,
   54-60
Geriatrics, 1-4
   departmental structure
      in, 3
Gout, 43
Great vessels, 12
Gynaecomastia, 72

Hallux valgus, 9
Hands
   claw deformity, 61
   osteoarthritis, 41
   rheumatoid arthritis, 42
   swan-neck deformity, 42
   wasting of small
      muscles, 61
Head injuries, 5, 22
Heart disorders, 45-7
Heberden's nodes, 41
Hemianopia, 17
Hemiplegia, 17, 18, 21
Hepatomegaly, 75
Hernias

hiatus, 56
post-operative incisional, 58
Herpes zoster, ophthalmic, 20
Hiatus hernia, 56
Hip, osteoarthritis, 42
Hyperostosis, 22, 40
Hypertension, 46
Hypotension, postural, 7
Hypothyroidism, 82

Ichthyosis, 68
Incontinence, urinary, 28-32
aetiology, 28
indwelling catheter, 32
local causes, 29
rash, 32
Infarction
cerebral, 14-16
embolic, 46
myocardial, 45
Intertrigo, submammary, 71
Intestine, obstruction, 60

Joint Disorders, 41-4

Keratosis, senile, 68
Knees
osteoarthritis, 41
pseudogout, 44

Legs, muscle disorders, 62-3
Lentigo maligna, 76
Liver enlargement, 75
Looser's zone, 37
Lungs
carcinoma, 50, 52
infections, 50-1, 53

Lupus erythematosus, 51, 64

Malnutrition, 54, 56
Melanoma, malignant, 76
Meningioma, 22
Motor neurone disease, 62
Mouth disorders, 54-6
Muscles
disorders, 61-5
spasticity, 63
wasting, 61-2
weakness, 64
Myasthenia gravis, 63
Myeloma, multiple, 40
Myxoedema, 82

Neoplasms, 72-7
see also carcinoma

Oedema
feet, 7
lymphatic, arm, 74
Oesophagus
achalasia, 65
stricture, 57
Onychogryphosis, 80
Osteoarthritis, 41-2
Osteomalacia, 33, 38
Osteoporosis, 33
spine, 36-7
Ovaries, carcinoma, 75

Paget's disease, 33, 38-9
Pancreas, carcinoma, 58
Paralysis, stroke and, 17, 18
Parkinsonism, falls in, 5
Pelvis
metastatic carcinoma, 73

Paget's disease, 39
Pemphigoid, 70
Pemphigus vulgaris, 71
Pneumothorax, 52
Polymyalgia rheumatica, 64
Polymyositis, 64
Pressure sores, 25-7, 32
Prostate
    carcinoma, 72
    hypertrophy, 31
Pruritus, 67
Pseudogout, 44
Psoriasis, 70
Ptosis, 63
    stroke and, 16
Purpura, 66, 82

Rheumatoid arthritis, 42

Scabies, 69
Schmorl's node, 36
Scleroderma, 65
Shoulder
    frozen, 65
    polymyalgia
        rheumatica, 64
Skin
    atrophy, 66
    disorders, 66-71
    neoplasms, 76-7
    wrinkling, 66
Skull
    acromegaly, 83
    hyperostosis, 22, 40
    multiple myeloma, 40
    Paget's disease, 39
Spine
    cervical, arthritis, 5, 8
    kyphosis, 36

osteoporosis, 36-7
Stomach, carcinoma, 57, 72
Stomatitis, angular, 56
Strokes, 11-18, 21
    complications, 11
Sway, backward, 5, 9

Telangiectasia, 64
Thrombocytopenia, 82
Thrombosis
    abdominal aorta, 48
    deep venous, 48
Thyrotoxicosis, 84
Tibia
    bowing, 38
    fracture, 37
Toenails, overgrown, 80
Transient ischaemic
    attacks (TIAs), 13-14
Tuberculosis, miliary, 53

Ulcers, diabetic, 83
Urethra, caruncle, 29
Urine
    retention, 31
    see also incontinence
Uterovaginal prolapse, 30

Varicose veins, 7
Vascular disease,
    peripheral, 47
Vertebral bodies,
    fractures, 37
Vision, strokes and, 14, 17

Warts, seborrhoeic, 68
Wrist
    fracture, 10
    rheumatoid arthritis, 42

WITHDRAWN FROM
A.E.C.C. LIBRARY

ANGLO-EUROPEAN COLLEGE OF CHIROPRACTIC